Olivia,

To the love of my life. You are a very old soul, the adversity has given you a deep well to pull from. With equal lightness to pull the "LIGHT" that can only come from Christ, Shine Bright, you were called to impact your generation.

Love Always,
Mom

11-16-2017

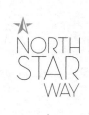

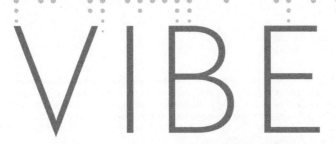

VIBE

Unlock the Energetic Frequencies
of Limitless Health, Love & Success

ROBYN OPENSHAW

NORTH STAR WAY

New York   London   Toronto   Sydney   New Delhi

NORTH
STAR
WAY

North Star Way
An Imprint of Simon & Schuster, Inc.
1230 Avenue of the Americas
New York, NY 10020

First North Star Way hardcover edition October 2017

NORTH STAR WAY and colophon are trademarks of Simon & Schuster, Inc.

For information about special discounts for bulk purchases, please contact Simon & Schuster Special Sales at 1-866-506-1949 or business@simonandschuster.com.

The North Star Way Speakers Bureau can bring authors to your live event.
For more information or to book an event, contact the North Star Way Speakers Bureau at 1-212-698-8888 or visit our website at www.thenorthstarway.com.

Interior design by Jaime Putorti

Manufactured in the United States of America

10 9 8 7 6 5 4 3 2 1

Library of Congress Cataloging-in-Publication Data

Names: Openshaw, Robyn.
Title: Vibe : unlock the energetic frequencies of limitless health, love & success / Robyn Openshaw.
Description: First Hardcover Edition. | New York : North Star Way, 2017.
Identifiers: LCCN 2017021660 (print) | LCCN 2017035970 (ebook) | ISBN 9781501163296 (ebook) | ISBN 9781501163289 (hardback)
Subjects: LCSH: Emotions. | Nutrition. | Self-care, Health. | BISAC: HEALTH & FITNESS / Healthy Living. | HEALTH & FITNESS / Nutrition. | HEALTH & FITNESS / Alternative Therapies.
Classification: LCC BF511 (ebook) | LCC BF511 .O66 2017 (print) | DDC 646.7--dc23
LC record available at https://lccn.loc.gov/2017021660

ISBN 978-1-5011-6328-9
ISBN 978-1-5011-6329-6 (ebook)

If you want to find the secrets of the universe, think
in terms of energy, frequency, and vibration.

—NIKOLA TESLA

: : : : :

Everything in life is vibration.

—ALBERT EINSTEIN

CONTENTS

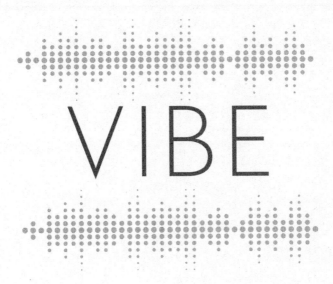

VIBE

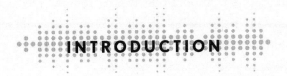

INTRODUCTION

The Great Vibration Discovery

Do you want in on the secrets of the universe?

I mean it. Do you?

There's a force field around you. *And you can feel it.*

Albert Einstein said, "Everything in life is vibration." Every atom in every molecule oscillates and is in motion and can be measured spectroscopically.

In Einstein's time, we couldn't yet measure electrical fields around a living thing. Now we can. In fact, science can measure the strong effect on your brain waves of the frequencies my heart is emitting if I'm in your energy field!

And there are other subtle energy fields that science can measure the effect of but can't yet pin down and "see."

Even thoughts, feelings, and other intangibles are simply energies.

When I began reading about energetic frequencies several years ago, I dove in and started to research, excited about the possibilities of this perfect organizing concept by which to measure literally everything we eat, think, do, feel, and say.

The thoughts we choose to spend our time on, the ways we react to stressors in our work and our lives in general, the foods we eat, and the substances we use to treat symptoms—they all have a measurable, demonstrable effect on our electrical and electromagnetic energies, or "vibration."

These choices affect our vibration—which, in turn, defines the kind of day we have, the quality of our professional work, and even the richness of our relationships and the quantity and quality of love we have to offer others.

And more: smoothing our vibrations heals the immune system, clears the mind, increases stress-reducing hormones such as DHEA, and decreases high-stress hormones such as cortisol, as documented by studies at the HeartMath Institute.

Everyone should understand how to raise their vibration. But while many have heard vague references to the concept, very few know what that means or how to do it.

In this book, I will show you how the vibrations of metabolizing your emotions; carefully chosen music, light, water, words, and other people; grounding outdoors; and plant-based medicinal substances and plant-based foods can completely change the energies of your life. Put simply, your small, daily choices are affecting whether you're living at high frequencies or experiencing chronically low oscillations!

Vibration is a trending topic—think of how often you hear someone refer to whether they like someone's "vibe" or say they're "resonating" or "vibing" with an idea presented to them. But most of us use this vocabulary with little knowledge of its origin or its power in our lives. I believe we can change the world with our understanding and use of it.

"Vibration" has its roots in the discoveries of the great Serbian scientist Nikola Tesla. During his lifetime, Tesla garnered some three hundred patents worldwide and discovered that absolutely everything has electrical frequency, or vibrational energy.

I have a cherry-red Tesla Model S in my garage, not just because I geek out about everything related to this hero of mine, Nikola Tesla, and his modern-day counterpart leading the charge, Elon Musk, and not only because the car is fast and sexy—but also because electric cars are a dream for many of us who envision sustainable life on earth for our grandchildren.

I want to decrease my carbon footprint and also be a part of raising the vibration of the planet, starting with helping you right now, today.

The visionary Elon Musk gave credit where credit was due and didn't name the car the Musk. He named it after a man who spent his entire life chasing energy, starting with a long journey across the ocean on a boat, where he was robbed of all but two pennies in his pocket.

Before he landed on US soil, Tesla dreamed of channeling Niagara Falls for energy, even though he'd never been to this continent or seen the great waterfalls. (Interestingly, others would later say that Niagara Falls is the only place on earth that fills the entire sonic spectrum—sound, light, water.) He accomplished that, making the falls an energy source for human needs, within a decade of arriving on our shores.

Like so many other scientific geniuses, he was better at innovating than he was shrewd in his business dealings—and he never achieved significant financial compensation for the astonishing discoveries that others made millions from.

One of the most earth-shattering findings of his lifetime was the fact that all matter has vibrational energy, or electrical frequency. That is, we are all electrical beings, made up of rapidly vibrating cells. Every atom in the universe oscillates at varying speeds.

Many people, I assume, are vaguely familiar with this concept. After all, there are some songs in the popular culture about it. To test that out, I asked my Facebook audience on the Green Smoothie Girl page: "What does high vibration mean to you?"

Here are some of the answers I got:

- "Does it have anything to do with our frequency?" —Angela S.
- "It means your energy vibration in connection to the universe."—Cindy H.
- "Marky Mark and the Funky Bunch—'It's such a good vibration! Such a sweet sensation!'"—Laura J.
- "Everything has a vibrational frequency. The healthiest foods have the highest frequencies."—Kathy S.
- "Sitting on my 'personal massager'?"—Shirley K.
- "A lot of movement?"—Lauren B.
- "Someone who is able to send good vibes to the people around them? No clue."—Toni H.
- "Harnessing the energy provided by eating living food, clean air, clean water, and sunshine!"—Patricia S.
- "It means powerful vibrations from an earthquake: tremor, shaking, and quaking."—Stephanie K.

Regardless of whether people have the vaguest notion about what "vibration" is, they don't know what powerful implications this has for their every choice, every day:

- Which foods you eat
- How much water you drink (and what's in that water)
- What you use to medicate yourself when you feel unwell
- What you think about while you're in the car or the shower
- What words you choose as you express yourself
- What emotions you spend your time indulging in—and what you do with them once you feel them
- What your risk of disease is
- How you feel in any given moment

- What your possibility for happiness is
- What you're attracting, in terms of other people, opportunities, and events

That, in short, is the power of vibration. You will learn in these pages about what I will call your Vibrational Quotient, or ViQ, which is nothing less than your health-and-happiness meter. We'll learn what it is, why it matters, and how to radically increase your own ViQ for the quality of life you may have dreamed of but have never known how to achieve.

I'm going to share a quiz with you, so you know what point you're starting from. Wherever you are right now, there's every possibility of increasing your ViQ dramatically by the time we're done!

Everything in the field of wellness, and even personal growth, can and should revolve around the basic, easily understood concept that every single thing we choose to eat—and everything we choose to think, feel, and do—lowers or raises our vibration.

And this makes all the difference in whether we can accomplish our destiny on this planet.

The rate and pitch of your own vibration dictate the level of your creativity, your physical and emotional health, and even your ability to love. Thus, raising your vibration is the key to rising above circumstances to achieve a life beyond your wildest dreams!

I know this because I have learned it, acted on it, and achieved it. I will share the devastated, low place from which I started—and what happened as I carried out each piece we'll be exploring along the path.

Frequency is not just an abstract scientific concept. It is extremely well documented in the field of physics, in part because of the advent of the electron microscope, which allows us to study subatomic particles in motion, or energies.

Examining vibrations and energies has massive, powerful implications for any human being's achievement of his or her purpose during a lifetime—implications, in fact, for the future viability of the human species in general.

Living at a consistently high and strong frequency, eventually you are achieving your own divine purpose, you're capable of a higher moral code, and self or ego becomes less important than purpose and connection and honoring every living being.

Living at 528 hertz (Hz), in fact—the frequency of love, of green things, of the core of the universe—is as close to the holy grail, or the ultimate human state of being, as we may ever get.

I have become highly attuned to high and low frequencies; chaotic, fractured frequencies; and strong and steady frequencies—and you can become so too. You're probably more attuned than you think.

Have you ever walked into a room, and even though the two people in it aren't speaking, you can tell by the charge in the room that they've just had an argument?

You've surely had the feeling when you interact with someone that you just can't get enough of them, and you find yourself seeking them out, asking their opinion, and inviting them to your home. And you've had the opposite experience, where you can't get away from someone fast enough because of dissonant energetic frequencies.

For that reason alone, you'll want to tune in to how we all respond to frequencies. If the uplevelers on this planet can sense yours, decode it, and decide without even thinking whether they want to work with you or not—well, we'd all better pay attention.

This is now measurable by electronic devices such as the electrocardiograph, which produces an ECG (electrocardiogram) that can show the impact on your heart waves or brain waves when someone in your energy field, touching you or even within a few feet of you, is emitting vibrations that carry emotions such as gratitude, lust, anger, compassion, or shame. Each has a specific vibration.

Let me show you very graphically how powerful frequencies can be. The following image shows two electrocardiograms, covering

200 seconds each, of a person experiencing anger (*top*), and a person experiencing deep gratitude (*bottom*).

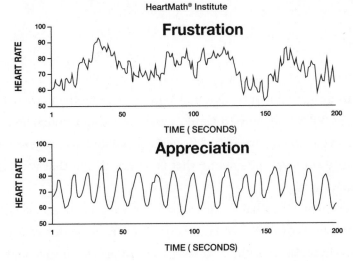

Heart-Rhythm Pattern of An Individual
HeartMath® Institute

I don't even have to use words to explain these graphics to you—just by looking, you know which of these two 200-second snapshots of frequencies *feels wonderful* and which one *feels awful*.

I will teach you how to "tune in." And how to shift from those awful-feeling frequencies to the beautiful ones.

We know from color, light, words, water, music, medicine, and science that vibration is real and that it has everything to do with your health—and more: your happiness.

Developing this valuable energetic intuition and awareness will make your relationships more grounded, more honest, and more rewarding. It will enhance your ability to do any kind of professional work and to communicate with more clarity and power.

The principles you'll learn here have the power to literally vibrate toxins out of your cells, allowing your cells to soak up nutrition more efficiently and to heal and become more disease resistant.

In fact, what you'll learn here is the very key to the Law of Attraction—attracting far more of the good and less of the bad into your life in every way.

:::: VIBRATIONAL QUOTIENT: :::: YOUR PERSONAL VIQ

What needs to be explored and brought to public consciousness is how to design your own Optimal Vibrational Quotient (what I'll refer to as ViQ) and how to think, every day, about your choices related to your electromagnetic frequency. I will talk to you about it in language you can understand, that is practical, and that you can experiment with.

Experiment with what you learn here until you know very clearly how magical it is to be fully conscious of your energetics at every moment—but also, over the next year, you can develop a sustainable lifestyle of powerful, grounded, high-quality energies.

Energetics is a science infused with art and beauty, and it is deeply meaningful and personal for anyone who is fortunate enough to discover it. It is about limitless potential, and it begins with the very fundamentals of all matter.

In this book, we will explore how earth's magnetics and energetics are increasing, and what the exciting implications of this are for human beings.

Even "dead" things are alive. Not to be morbid, but let's say you went to a morgue and pulled out a drawer containing a three-day-old corpse and cut off a tiny chunk of skin. You're already cringing, but bear with me—this is interesting.

Let's say you put that skin under a high-powered microscope. What would you see?

You might think you would just see stillness. Objects, cells . . . motionless.

But you wouldn't see that at all. You would see motion. That's right, even dead flesh is in motion. (Of course, the cells of the corpse are vibrating at much lower frequencies than yours are.) If they weren't in motion, how would that corpse eventually become dust?

All matter is in motion and is energetically vibrating. Every cell of your body. Since each cell participates in, or is part of, a specific organ, the organ's vibration also has a specific frequency, which can be measured.

And that organ contributes to your overall vibration, which can also be measured. You contribute to the energetic fields of the people within three feet of you—and those electromagnetic, electrical, and other subtle-energy fields are real, documentable, whirling masses of electrons in oscillating motion.

It's possible to measure frequency in cycles per nanosecond. Few people do measure this or publicize it to us, which is a tragedy. We're too busy measuring the cycles of planets around the sun, or the velocity per second of a vehicle, or the temperature of a substance—or the caloric value of food or the grams of proteins, fats, and carbs in it.

We have lots of metrics in our lives, but the one that blows away all the others is mostly ignored. So many different measurements we're preoccupied with—yet you, reading this, have no idea what your current frequency is, in hertz or any other unit of measure, let alone your Optimal ViQ.

Somehow, a very powerful measurement that affects all of us constantly isn't considered or described in applied food science or the medical science that the average person encounters.

But just thinking about electrical frequency can transform the way you see human beings, the world, and your own potential in that world.

::::: SO, LET'S GET THE VIBE GOING :::::

In all the work that has been done on the science of vibration and energy, there has been extensive focus on intuition and spirituality and how our thoughts become our reality. But while we will not neglect these things, we are going to start at the very beginning.

We're taking the goal of increasing your vibration to the very foundation—to the fuel you choose every day as food, to the thoughts you have and what you do with them, to what you spend your free time doing. All of that affects the energies of your every cell!

After all, if you drive a Mercedes, you don't put the lowest-grade fuel in your car at the gas pump. Every thoughtful Mercedes driver chooses the high-grade fuel. Anything less is insanity, because you don't put inferior fuel in a $90,000 car.

I'll discuss how the ways we've been trained to measure food value are fairly useless and fabricated by profit-driven industries. There's a new way to look at food that is easy to understand and can revolutionize the way you see your food choices every day. It may not be what the food industry uses to measure food values, but it's valid and important.

To this end, I'm going to give you a 7-Day Detox menu, which will show you what's possible. Do it with me, and your mind will be blown as you connect the dots between your symptoms, mood, and overall vibration and what you eat, think, and do on a daily basis.

And it just might be the missing link to kick your cravings and addictions to the curb once and for all. Understanding energetic frequencies will change the way you see your diet and your motivations to eat specific kinds of foods.

Once you achieve this, you'll never go back to feeling the way you've always felt. You'll protect your high vibe, as I have.

When you understand these beautiful concepts as they unfold in these pages, you will see yourself as having far more potential than you've considered before. What you learn can transform your thoughts, feelings, and vocabulary, as well as your perspective on what you are capable of.

The rate of your entire being's vibration dictates the level of your creativity, your physical and emotional health, and even your ability to love. Thus, raising your vibration is the key to rising above circumstances to achieve a life you may have quit dreaming about long ago.

Once you understand what a high-vibration life is, you won't settle for anything less!

So, here's the secret to health: it's all about vibration. It's about choosing foods, medicines, and practices that raise your vibration and help you discover your Optimal ViQ.

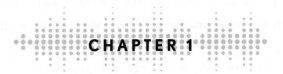

CHAPTER 1

How Raising Your Vibrational Quotient Will Radically Change Your Life

::::: FUNDAMENTALS OF VIBRATION :::::

Before we dive in, you should understand five basic scientific concepts about why a cell, a substance, a thought, or a human being has a certain vibration.

Vibrations can be felt (such as earthquake tremors), seen (light waves), and heard (sound waves). What we register with our senses is just a fraction of the frequencies all around us!

For instance, the human ear can hear about ten octaves of the audio spectrum, but you can purchase an inexpensive dog whistle and blow it and hear nothing—but dogs can hear it, and they'll come running. Elephants and moles can hear frequencies well below the lowest register you can hear. And whales, dolphins, and bats can hear pitches in the ultrasonic range higher than we can.

When the range of sound frequencies increases to the top of the spectrum, they eventually become light. And there are vibrations of light that are invisible to the human eye, because colors have "octaves" as well—and as they change hue when frequency increases, eventually there is nothing but brilliant white light, which some believe is God's frequency.

As with many other things—such as the fact that as much as 90 percent of your body mass is actually not your "body" (most of "you" is stuff that doesn't contain your DNA, such as fluids and bacterial organisms)—you severely limit yourself if you think that the only reality is the reality that you see, hear, and understand.

This is the fundamental premise of Einstein's physics and his revolutionary $E=mc^2$, which eventually led to the burgeoning field of quantum physics. Prior to Max Planck, Einstein, and others "breaking" Newtonian physics, scientific thought assumed that the world was made up of machinations, parts, and processes. The prevailing belief was that a body and the forces acting upon it, through the laws of motion, explained phenomena around the universe.

What has evolved since that split in the theory of all matter has given rise to applications like superconducting magnets, lasers and magnetic resonance imaging in medicine, electron microscopy, semiconductors, and an understanding of many physical and biological phenomena.

We are discussing the application of the principles discovered in quantum physics to nothing less essential and nothing less personal than whether you are healthy and happy.

So let's start with five basic principles you must understand before we dive in.

1. Everything in the Universe Is Energy

You may not think of the piece of furniture you're looking at or sitting on as energy, but it is. Your breath is energy. Your fingernail is energy. Even a rock is energy. But thoughts and emotions and your connection to another human being or an animal—all these are energy too. In fact, you are made of the same energies that can be found in various places around the universe, but these energies have come together in the very special, one-of-a-kind form that is uniquely you!

2. You Have a Vibrational Quotient

You don't have something like a Fitbit on your wrist or a mood ring on your finger as your vibration barometer. But you should. Because when you are vibrating at a high frequency, you are more likely to achieve everything on your to-do list today, or get a raise this month, or—if you live this way consistently and sustainably—finish a PhD and write an award-winning book in the next five years. Or whatever your big, hairy, audacious goal is!

When you vibrate at a high frequency, you are more likely to find a high-quality partner and love that partner, and others you choose, deeply and long-term, with patience and tolerance. You're more likely to be at peace with that person's quirks and choices, even the ones that affect you.

You are more likely to feel celebratory and uplifted daily when encountering small positives in your environment, such as a baby's laugh or a pretty sunrise, and you're unlikely to experience long-term states of depression or anxiety.

When the ViQ measuring device that we're imagining says you're vibrating high and strong, you aren't set back by the things that don't go your way. You are patient, thorough, and completely captivated by your projects and tasks in that amazing flow state where you lose track of time and nothing matters but the excitement of unfolding a pattern of your creative process—whether you direct a choir, play tennis, or design circuit boards for a living.

When your vibration is high, your cells are multiplying, dividing, and carrying out their purposes perfectly for their full life span until they become obsolete and die a natural cell death—rather than crawling slowly along in the bloodstream, deprived of oxygen, in an acidic medium, dying prematurely or mutating into cancer cells that take over healthy functions.

When your electrical energy is optimal, you are likely to go out like a light bulb when life is over—rather than fade on the long, painful, slow dimmer switch of the suffering, low-vibration human being.

3. Like Attracts Like

Your energetic vibration, like a magnet, actually attracts similar frequencies. So, when a low-vibration human being who is ill mentally, spiritually, and physically encounters another person of approximately the same electrical frequency, they are literally attracted to each other.

This is often called the Law of Attraction, and it is a law of physics with its roots in the discoveries of Tesla.

Similarly—and this is an exciting concept for your future, once you've read this book—a high-vibration human being whose discourse is about creative ideas, literally buzzing with electric energy, a person who imagines positive outcomes and seeks out high frequencies in his or her activities, friends, and feelings, attracts other human beings vibrating at the same frequencies.

A person making high-frequency choices attracts high-quality opportunities and people, and even money! For instance, people who opt into high frequencies as a lifestyle have the enviable problem of always trying to figure out which of the many wonderful opportunities before them to focus on. Others, chronically vibrating at low oscillations, can't find a job.

4. A Substance with a Higher Frequency Can Cause the Vibration of a Lower-Frequency Substance to Increase

This principle has exciting, important implications for your emotional, spiritual, mental, and physical health. If having high-vibration substances in your energy field raises yours, then knowledge about what those substances are (and which are the low-vibration ones) can change your life, just through awareness and tiny, easy choices every day.

The people in the room you're in, the electronic devices in your energy field, the substances you put on your skin, and the food you swallow all affect your vibration—often dramatically. We will give many examples of this.

5. There Is an Opposite to the Law of Entropy

You probably learned in high school physics that the universe moves from order to disorder. However, it is a fascinating counterpoint that *human beings can, and often do, ascend to higher and higher states of vibration.*

While many of their peers are sliding backward into lower frequencies, there are people who, by American standards, are significantly "aging"—all of them over the age of fifty-five—who continue to increase what they give to the world. These are examples you might know, and they are among my heroes: Oprah Winfrey, Tony Robbins, Dr. Daniel Amen, Arianna Huffington, Dr. Peter Diamandis, Bono, Anne Lamott, Richard Branson, Dr. Gabriel Cousens, Bob Proctor, Jimmy Carter, Deepak Chopra, Louise Hay, Marianne Williamson, Byron Katie, and the Dalai Lama.

Recently there has been an exciting discovery that contradicts our tendency to think that the world is going to hell in a handbasket. In fact, there are exciting implications for human beings of the scientific discovery that our earth has actually been increasing in frequency in recent years!

We've discussed the principle of quantum physics that something of a higher frequency can cause the vibration of something with a lower frequency to increase—so the point here is that you have the momentum of the ground underneath you, the very polarity of the axis of the planet, to assist your own upleveling!

: : : : :

You can improve the quality of your career, your mood, your physical health, your intimate partner, your family life, and more—

simply by learning and applying the concepts we will explore in these pages.

When we're functioning at low vibrations, we have repetitive negative thoughts that hijack more productive things that could be happening in our brains. We attract negative people, events, dramas, and addictive activities into our lives. We can't figure out why other people do what they do, and we can't seem to get out of their orbit, so we feel victimized by them. We aren't in tune with others' vibrations because our own are thick, heavy, and slow—so we tend to make poorer choices in relationships, career, and life.

We often run out of steam, and we live as if under a dark, heavy cloud. Life is challenging, and we're more prone to depression. We feel we're stuck at the bottom of the pile or fighting our way out of being lost in the middle of a crowd. As one thing goes wrong, like dominoes in a row, more and more things go wrong—you lose your job, the electricity bill doesn't get paid, the power gets shut off . . . you get the idea.

But when we operate at higher frequencies, we think positive thoughts, we're often optimistic and excited, and we attract positive people, events, activities, and outcomes. Life is much smoother than for our low-vibration neighbors, without the mood "crashes"—and while things may occasionally go wrong, we course correct quickly because we're clear and healthy in our thoughts, intuitive and mindful in our relationships, creative in our work, and at peace in the world.

We tend to enjoy the day, sleep well, and look forward to the future. We shine, we are at the top of our game often, and we view setbacks as temporary and as helpful life lessons. As one, two, three high-quality individuals seek us out, others see that, and they want to work with us, date us, or befriend us too. One promotion after another leads to directorships or executive-level jobs—and headhunters giving us a call periodically, just in case we're available.

These are simply examples of the trajectory and momentum of energies: negatives beget more negatives, and positives beget more positives.

But I want to share my own story that led me to writing this book in the first place.

::::: MY STORY: :::::
FROM LOW VIBE TO HIGH VIBE

Long before I discovered the Law of Attraction (to which I originally had a very negative reaction) and the science of Nikola Tesla, I personally was living a very low-vibration life. And I was only in my twenties. Wasn't that supposed to be the prime of my life, my youth?

From age eighteen to twenty-eight, I was eating the standard American diet. I didn't get fat overnight. It was long and slow, so gradual that I hardly noticed the decline in any given month. Two years out of college, three years after my wedding, I was thirty pounds overweight and working a desk job, and I never felt very healthy. (Later, with pregnancy, I would gain even more weight and hit a high of 206 pounds.)

These were the daily features of my life. I call it:

My Low-Vibration Life (My Twenties)

1. I didn't move my body much. On the occasions I walked for a mile, I was exhausted. I suffered. I avoided playing the sports I'd always loved.

2. I never wanted to do anything or go anywhere. A family vacation seemed overwhelming—the planning, the uncertainty, and what if I had no energy when I got there? So we didn't go.

3. The natural ambition I was born with was greatly diminished, if not gone. I'd earned an advanced degree and written a book while I was young. But all my drive had disappeared into an energetic black hole.

4. My little kids probably wished somebody else was their mom. I was moody and impatient.

5. I got every little virus that went around. Sometimes worse: strep, requiring antibiotics. One winter, I was sick ten times!

6. I rarely wanted to have sex. It took too much energy. And here I was, at the age when everyone is supposed to be having sex like rabbits! This wasn't helpful to my relationship with my husband.

7. All I wanted to do was sleep, eat, and watch TV. Most days, that's about all I did. (Unsurprisingly, these are the lowest-vibration activities humans engage in.)

8. Any negative event, no matter how small, would tip me over emotionally. A small argument with my husband could put me into a crying jag.

9. I spent a lot of time thinking and talking about my childhood of abuse and trauma, as well as other negative events in the past.

You may relate to my story. After all, it describes most of America.

Fortunately, even in that very low state, I began to discover some exciting truths that would radically transform my life. They were so exciting, as absolutely everything in my life began to change for the better, that I wanted to tell others about them.

Once you put even one of the things I'll teach you in this book into practice, you'll begin energetic momentum, and each subsequent action you take gets easier and easier! (Remember the law of physics that bodies in motion tend to stay in motion. And the corollary: that bodies at rest tend to stay at rest. So taking a first step is important, and it gets something very exciting going.)

I don't have to convince you that every day I count on the high-vibration features of my life mentioned in the list below, because you can imagine I wouldn't commit to an eighty-eight-city speaking tour in 2014 while raising four kids by myself and running a company with fifteen employees if I couldn't depend on strong energy, mood, and health.

And it's not that I have a perfect diet, because I don't. (Who does?) It's that I've discovered what matters most: the types of foods to eat every day in ways that work for me. And I focus on that.

Most of us are completely confused about what the absolute essentials are in nutrition and wellness, because there is so much noise out there, with all the food cults and marketing and new diets competing for attention.

I'm about to share with you the amazing features of my life I count on every single day, after fifty trips around the sun. The life I'm about to describe characterized the entire decade of my forties and now continues into my fifties. And I know how to maintain it.

I feel far, far better than I did when I was twenty-five, half my life ago. And I call this:

My High-Vibration Life (My Forties and Fifties)

- I play competitive sports, have advanced in tennis ratings three times in my forties to the level of 4.0, and run five miles most mornings. All of it *gives* me energy, rather than depleting it.
- I have tons of energy. I don't measure it, ration it, dole out small quantities—I count on it and I plan and execute ambitious things.

- I need less sleep—six hours a night is great.
- I'm always up for an adventure, especially travel. Hiking, skiing, a yoga weekend? I'm in!
- I wake up excited about my day, making lists, dreaming up plans for my business or my next trip with the kids or my friends.
- I have an even temperament, no emotional crashes, no PMS, no rage.
- I have positive and fun relationships with my kids and others.
- My libido is what it should have been in my twenties.
- Setbacks in life don't tip me over—even though I've had all the "big ones" hit me in my forties, including divorce and other tough stuff.
- I'm far more capable of solving problems, so I make bigger, bolder goals.
- I can't even imagine watching TV. I have too many more interesting things on my bucket list.

What would *your* high-vibration life look like? Do you dare to dream about it?

Dream about it with me. Start by wanting it.

You may be thinking: She's talking to everyone but me. I'm too far gone. Everything hurts, I'm far more than the thirty pounds overweight she mentioned earlier, and I can't even remember feeling good. I'm exhausted, and I'm on all kinds of pills and can't even count the diagnoses doctors have given me.

No, I *am* talking to you. You're *not* reading the wrong book. You're *not* too far gone. I wrote this book precisely *for* you—and I'm about to tell you something I think will excite you and give you some inspiration.

That's all I need—for a spark to light. I can work with that. If you don't yet believe the high-vibration life I've just described is pos-

sible for you, that's okay. Just keep reading. It's probably because you haven't experienced it in a very long time, or maybe ever. You've had moments, though—glimpses of it.

You know something of what high, beautiful energy is, from way back. Remember running a race in elementary school, where you felt you were flying and passing everyone else? Have you experienced moments, even hours, of "pure grace," when everything in the world felt right and peaceful and your work and your efforts all fell into place with ease?

Have you ever experienced sheer, unadulterated love and awe toward another human being, with no expectations, demands, or resentment—just love?

If you're not yet in the zone of hoping for, requiring, and attracting pure high vibrations in your life, I will carry us both, at this moment in time. I will hope for it, and believe in it, for you! I believe *your high-vibration life* is possible and just around the corner.

Increasing your Vibrational Quotient (ViQ) is our goal: between now and when you finish reading this book, and in completing the 7-Day Detox journey.

My job here is to show you that it is the result of small, consistent daily choices—and the radical reboot we're going to accomplish in just one week, giving you a taste of what's possible!

Now, if a few moments ago you resonated with that idea of "No, it's too late for me—I'm too ill or I'm too old," you simply must read this:

Do you know what your liver does for you? How many ways does it serve you?

Would it shock you to learn that scientists who study human physiology estimate that the liver has somewhere between five hundred and a thousand functions in the human body?

Wow. If you have a liver (and I'm fairly certain you do), take a minute to thank it. Tell it. Put your hands on it, right below the left

side of your rib cage. It's okay, no one's looking. That incredible organ gets so little praise from you, so it's long past due:

"Thank you, liver, for all the ways you serve me!"

Be in awe of your liver for a minute. Even while you're asleep, your liver is working. It's actually completely filtering your entire blood supply every four minutes! Isn't that incredible?

And here's what's even more exciting: Did you know that you will replace every single cell of your liver within the next ninety days?

It's true.

If your liver does at least five hundred things for you, do you think there could be a difference in the way you look—or the way you feel—if you built your *next* liver out of different materials? Better materials? High-vibration materials?

Three months from now, you can and will essentially have a brand-new liver. Do you think there's a difference in the way a liver performs if it is built from corn chips and diet soda versus, perhaps, homemade green smoothies, for example?

It's something to think about. You can have dramatic results and you can have them fast. You can't have them if snack cakes and cola are what you fill your cart with on your next trip to the grocery store. You may not get those dramatic results if you aren't willing to give up a little bit of TV time for some vibration-raising self-care.

But it's exciting to think that you can be, in literally hundreds of ways, a brand-new you in just three months.

::::: THE LAW OF ATTRACTION :::::

When I watched the cult movie *The Secret* many years ago, I was less than impressed. In fact, I rolled my eyes and told everyone who ever brought it up how dumb I thought it was.

As with many things, I didn't understand it at first. I still have some of the same reactions to it that I did then, even though later my studies of frequencies made the Law of Attraction a realistic, proven, and very valuable principle to me.

One of my main negative reactions was that if one did not fully understand the Law of Attraction, one might watch the movie and reduce this important principle to "wishful thinking." Or, in the words of religion, there's a danger of the film becoming advocacy for "faith without works." I rolled my eyes at the thought that I could drive into the Wal-Mart parking lot and "manifest" to get a front-row parking spot rather than one far away from the entrance. (Which was, I recall, one of the examples used in the movie.)

I don't need to find a front-row parking spot every time, and my sometimes overly analytical mind went to: "But what about all the other people who didn't get the front-row spot because I did?"

Also, I don't believe that a million bucks is going to fall out of the sky and conk me on the head just because I wish it so. This was one of my gripes with how I felt the Law of Attraction was reduced or transmitted in the film.

It's a bit more complex than that, while also being rather elegantly simple. The fact is, when we have a positive thought, it makes a follow-up positive action 100 percent more likely—which then leads to the desired result. Now, that may be more boring than thinking you can squeeze your eyes shut and want, really a lot, to be a winner of the lottery, and it will magically happen.

And I thought it was farcical that someone might watch that movie and think, simplemindedly, that if a person just wants things enough, they will happen.

But wanting something enough truly does make that thing far more likely to happen. Intention is powerful, as proven by thousands of studies.

When I was twenty-two, I set the goal of being completely out of debt, including fully owning my home and a second home, and having enough money to have passive interest income finance a comfortable lifestyle. I did the math, and I knew how many millions of dollars I needed and how I'd have to invest them.

I set that goal because financial security is very important to me. "Stuff" and "things" aren't particularly interesting to me. Security against uncertainty, anxiety, and economic downturns are what fuel me.

I wanted it because I'd planned to work till I was old, regardless of whether I needed the money or not. I wasn't interested (I'm still not!) in living on a golf course or a beach and drinking margaritas all day—I wanted to do beautiful, meaningful work that blesses other people's lives, without worrying about whether it was making money. I wanted my last few decades to be about service and teaching the world, whoever would listen, what little bits of radical wisdom I'd achieved in my first fifty years. I wanted to spend more time and energy being the teacher I was born to be. (I am the eldest of eight children, and found ways to be a teacher, albeit a bossy one sometimes, from a very young age.)

But I didn't achieve this big financial goal only because I wished for it—and then sat at home watching TV and reading pulp fiction and eating doughnuts and wishing, wishing, wishing.

I achieved it because putting words to it, creating a high-frequency intention (focused energy), and reminding myself of it often fueled massive action for twenty-five years, leading up to the achievement of that goal after an epic amount of work.

I achieved it because of all the other energetically upleveling practices I learned along the way, which allowed me to tap my creative energies to become a success, despite major challenges including being a single mom for the past nine years.

The energies of choosing that very big goal were absolutely necessary to making that thing happen, that financial freedom that I'm sure almost everyone wants. It wasn't just a first step. It was the kero-sene that fueled my actions and education and all the steps along the way.

It took me more years than I had intended. My goal was to have all those investments in place, with sustainable interest income to finance my life, by age forty. I achieved the goal at forty-eight.

And, of course, now I have more goals.

As is normal, I had many setbacks along the way. Such as no ali-mony, no inheritance, and no investors—those advantages enjoyed by many who make their fortunes. Such as a divorce, which almost always sets people back financially. Such as kids going to college and needing cars and other things, and having to finance that without help from a partner. Such as a conflict with a billion-dollar company that caused the loss of income I'd spent two and a half years working for. Such as three different businesses failing over the years. Such as an employee stealing money from my company, and me losing money in investments and business partnerships. All of these pushed me backward, further from the goal, and required me to start over several times, to work hard, build something, trouble-shoot every day, and learn constantly.

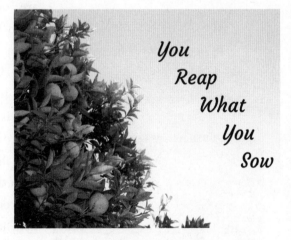

You Reap What You Sow

What you do with your life, whether you make something beautiful of it, absolutely must start with intention. There is also the Law of the Harvest that must follow the Law of Attraction.

That is, you reap what you sow.

But we will explore in depth how even the very worst things that happen to us translate into powerful, undeniable, grounded presence. Strength of character, you might say. I have been fascinated, my entire life, and have watched with keen interest how people prove who they are when in their darkest hour.

Recognize it as the energy in the right space at the right time, with a purpose that will reveal itself. Because occasionally a small but radical thought becomes a global movement that changes the course of life on this planet for the better.

And often a small thought can change your entire life. Because, after all, you don't become who you are despite your challenges. You become deep, wise, and, well, very literally, *because* of them.

:::: YOUR OPTIMAL VIQ ::::

Let's repeat the principle of quantum physics I shared with you earlier: a substance of a higher frequency can cause the vibration of a lower-frequency substance to increase.

High is one measurement, but *solid, grounded,* and *consistent* are other aspects—and if they seem mutually exclusive with *high* vibes, they're not. Sometimes you have to slow down to speed up. And there isn't just one frequency that is perfect for you at all times. There are creative frequencies, and there are lower, more peaceful resting frequencies—obviously, you don't want your brain firing with ideas at midnight in a high-frequency state. Alpha, beta, and theta states are all appropriate at different times.

People prove who they are in their darkest hour.

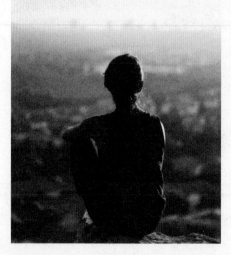

But the issue, then—without

getting particularly scientific, and perhaps grossly oversimplifying—is twofold: how *low* your frequencies are (the person who just can't get off the couch or is chronically angry or depressed), and how *chaotic* they are (the person who can't stay focused and who makes decisions based on the moment rather than his long-term best interests).

And those are our waking states. Of course, sometimes we don't enjoy peaceful, steady frequencies at night either.

Finding your Optimal ViQ and quickly turning around any downshifting frequencies, when needed, is a skill set. We're going to start with knowledge. But I'm also going to give you some very actionable, practical things you can do to keep your vibration high and consistent every day of your life starting—now!

::::: HOW HIGH IS YOUR VIBE? THE QUIZ! :::::

This quiz isn't intended to make you feel bad. In fact, one of the principles of your new life that taps greater energetics is to *observe* more often, not only to increase awareness but also to *decrease judgment*. So take this fourteen-question quiz to measure where you want your improvements to be—not to inflict more damage to your psyche with harsh self-judgment! My intent here is to give you benchmarks, to help you identify areas you want to focus on.

Answer each question honestly, and add up all the points—then let's evaluate what your total points indicate about the vibration of your life.

If you prefer to take an automatically scored test, you'll find it, as well as a Five-in-One Yogic Meditation and many other special gifts I've made to enhance your high-vibration life, at **GreenSmoothie Girl.com/VibeResources**. (Though I'll refer to the Resources page many times in this book, I won't repeat the URL, so mark and dog-ear this page!)

Rate the amount of each item in your life.

    1 = Rarely or Never

    2 = Less Than Daily or Occasionally

    3 = Often or Daily

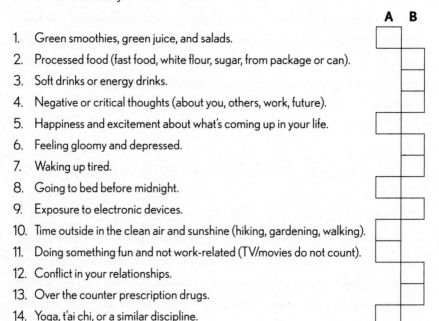

                                                             A   B

1. Green smoothies, green juice, and salads.
2. Processed food (fast food, white flour, sugar, from package or can).
3. Soft drinks or energy drinks.
4. Negative or critical thoughts (about you, others, work, future).
5. Happiness and excitement about what's coming up in your life.
6. Feeling gloomy and depressed.
7. Waking up tired.
8. Going to bed before midnight.
9. Exposure to electronic devices.
10. Time outside in the clean air and sunshine (hiking, gardening, walking).
11. Doing something fun and not work-related (TV/movies do not count).
12. Conflict in your relationships.
13. Over the counter prescription drugs.
14. Yoga, t'ai chi, or a similar discipline.

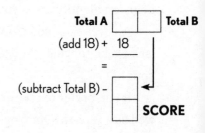

Total A ☐ ☐ **Total B**

(add 18) + 18

=

(subtract Total B) – ☐

☐ **SCORE**

22-28 points/High ViQ: You are making a great effort toward a high-quality life; others are likely noticing it and want to learn from you, be around you more. You're uplifting, and you're in a rare category of self-disciplined and happy people. We can always make improvements, and you're likely reading this book for even greater possibilities and to teach others. Good job—be a beacon to others, and continue your incremental improvement!

13-21 points/Moderate ViQ: You've already done some work in your life. You've still got some areas to work on, and you've come to the right place for that! Your low scores are areas to address, and the rest of this book is all about how to do that. You should be able to notice a remarkable difference in ViQ as you go through the 7-Day Detox, as well as the year of challenges following.

0-12 points/Low ViQ: You're probably less satisfied with your life than you could be, and you picked up this book because you want to attract more high vibrations in your life. The way to attract it is to become it, and you've got lots of ways to improve and climb a ladder to a life you may only dream of. You've also got the highest potential to really see a difference with every single practice you read about here, as well as doing the 7-Day Detox!

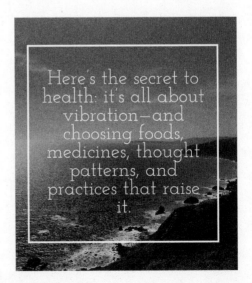

Here's the secret to health: it's all about vibration—and choosing foods, medicines, thought patterns, and practices that raise it.

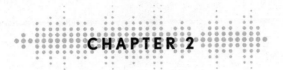

CHAPTER 2

Mindsets and Emotions:
How to Control Them for High Vibration

::::: THE MENTAL DISCIPLINE OF OPTIMAL VIQ :::::

This chapter is about mindfulness and choice in your thoughts and emotions. Learning to discipline your mind is every bit as important as eating nutrient-dense whole-plant foods. Getting a firm grasp on this can help you to never again be at the mercy of negative thinking and feeling.

How many books have you read that, besides making good dinner conversation, you didn't use to uplevel your life? Let's not let *this* book be like that!

Let's use this information you're gaining to get really clear with yourself, every day, about whether you're upleveling or downleveling your vibration as life moves on—toward your greatest contribution or toward declining contribution. It can happen almost imperceptibly. But right now you can ask yourself which one you are doing.

Are you on the long, slow decline? What we all love to call "aging"—but which is mostly unnecessary physical and mental decline?

If you feel like you're going downhill, it's not too late to turn that around. The actions you can take to nurture your physical and emo-

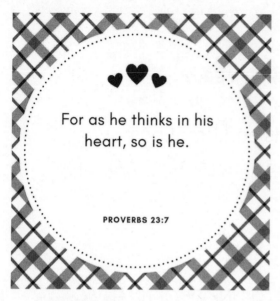

For as he thinks in his
heart, so is he.

PROVERBS 23:7

tional and mental health I have carefully curated in this book because they are so effective. They've all been key in turning my own life around, and there is published data on the power of each and every principle we're bringing to light in this course.

What I'm about to teach you will not be effective unless you're willing to let go of some possibly deeply held beliefs, even some elements of your identity. Are you open to that? To letting go of things that aren't serving you well?

Because depending on how you answer the next questions, you could absolutely change your life in ways that will be incredibly powerful, to turn a downward trajectory back upward.

Do you see yourself—be very honest right now, this is important—as a victim of circumstance, not in control of your life? Do you feel that bad things tend to happen to you?

If you're not sure, go to the Resources page and take the "locus of control" test, a short quiz developed by Julian B. Rotter in 1966. If you score at the low end, 0 to 5, you are a person who sees yourself as in control of your life. If you're at the high end, 9 to 13, you are someone who feels that fate or other people or forces outside your own control are captaining your ship.

Now, you might be responding:

It's not my fault I got cancer!

I couldn't help that my husband left me for my next-door-neighbor; I was a good wife!

I worked my guts out in my business, but it failed anyway!

I get it. Are you thinking something like this? What are your personal resistances?

If we were talking face-to-face, I'd smile and nod and validate you as you say things of this nature. And then I'd gently tell you that's not the point. At all. Remember: if you're over age forty, shit has happened to you. And I mean *serious shit* has happened to you.

To you, and me, and everyone else we know. (This is empirically easy to document; it's in a lot of published research.) And not all of it is our fault.

But what we do next is where the successes separate from the failures.

What do we do with the setbacks? Does the way you process your challenges in life, how you talk about them and how you use them after the fact in your conduct, increase your vibration and what you contribute in the world? Or does what you do with your challenges devastate your frequency and everyone else's around you?

What's clear, in research, is that whether we opt into success or not depends on whether we *believe that we influence the outcome.* Some key ideas:

- *Self-efficacy* refers to believing yourself capable of taking steps that will improve your situation. This belief is an important aspect of human motivation and behavior, and it influences the action (or inaction) to change your life.
- Self-efficacy affects your ability to learn, your motivation, and your performance. Usually we attempt to learn and perform only those things we believe we can be successful at.
- A major influence on decision making is the belief in personal relevance. When you believe that what you decide matters, you are more likely to make a decision (deciding whether or not to vote in an election, for instance).

- *Locus of control* describes the degree to which you perceive that outcomes result from your own behavior versus external forces. Those with an internal locus of control believe they alone are responsible for their own success (hard work, talent, decisions, personal attributes, etc.). Those with an external locus of control believe that external forces affect their life's outcomes (fate, luck, others' actions, etc.).

As Gandhi said:

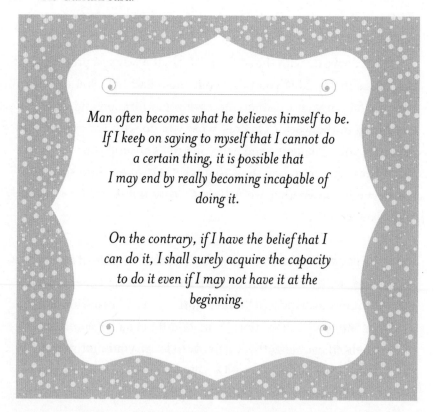

Man often becomes what he believes himself to be. If I keep on saying to myself that I cannot do a certain thing, it is possible that I may end by really becoming incapable of doing it.

On the contrary, if I have the belief that I can do it, I shall surely acquire the capacity to do it even if I may not have it at the beginning.

Do you control everything in your life? No.

Do you have control over more of it than you think? Likely yes.

Do you have to know the difference, where to spend your time and what to let go of? Of course you do.

But the biggest differentiator between successful and unsuccessful people, healthy people and unhealthy people, is . . .

The successful ones take action. They believe that what they do matters, that they can influence the outcome. They learn from their troubles; they move forward; they let go of trauma and release it into the universe with peace.

The unsuccessful ones are defeatist and see themselves at the mercy of others and the whims of circumstance.

Which one are you?

:::: CHECKING IN EVERY DAY: :::: WHAT'S THIS DOING TO MY VIBE?

People over the age of fifty-five are a great group to observe, if you care to look at vibrational quality of life. The choices they have made up to this point dictate whether they are upshifting, as a small minority of them are—bringing massive value to their families, to their communities, to the world—because of all this incredible life experience they have.

Look around. Most folks over fifty-five have shrinking lives on the decline; most of their talk centers on their problems and their physical ailments, and most of their free time is spent watching TV and engaging in low-vibration activities.

They are often found observing others living life (their grandchildren or people in the movies) instead of living it themselves. I'm not pointing this out to you to criticize them—I'm pointing this out because you're seeing it too, and it may not have occurred to you yet that you can opt out of that kind of downshifting. After all, seeing so much of it around us, we could easily just accept "aging" as the norm.

A good friend of mine—I'll call him Dan—recently flew to Europe to give two sold-out lectures. What he does for a living is truly changing the world, beyond his wildest dreams.

Like me, Dan unintentionally got a big fan base just by sharing his amazing sickness-to-health story online. Many years ago, he beat an often-deadly cancer through extraordinary holistic means, and he now shares the stories of others who have done the same. He researches and imparts little-known but powerful information on the Internet to an avid following.

Now he has the equivalent of four giant sold-out football stadiums full of people reading what he has to say every week in his newsletters, like I do.

This is how I think of my audience every time I sit down to write to all those of you who've been following me on GreenSmoothieGirl .com—that my readership could fill the university stadium near my house to capacity four times. It makes me a little breathless—and that's just the point: to remember that in every seat is a real, live person with dreams and with trauma, hoping that maybe I can help. As Peter Parker's uncle Ben wisely told him:

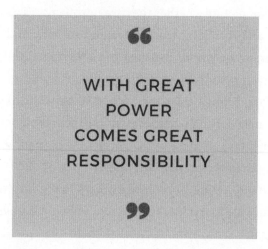

> **66**
>
> ## WITH GREAT POWER COMES GREAT RESPONSIBILITY
>
> **99**

My friend Dan feels the same way. I see him as a little brother, and I often tell him, "Don't forget—this 'reach' you've attained, thanks to the digital age, should not be taken for granted. It is a sacred trust. I hope you always do whatever benefits your audience, regardless of money. Because each one of them has hope in his or her heart when watching your video or reading your blog."

So Dan was at the airport one day on the way to Europe with both his parents, who are aging, and his father had a panic attack about flying and didn't get on the plane.

Dan went to Europe and gave two amazing talks. He was mobbed afterward by emotional, grateful people because his work has helped them turn their health around. He came home feeling that taking his message to another continent was one of the most exciting and rewarding experiences of his life.

And his father missed it.

Let me ask you: Are you okay with the fact that you may live with such significant low vibrations—fear, illness, or hate—that you miss out on the greatest things happening for your child in your lifetime?

I absolutely understand that aging will eventually happen to all of us, and that not everything that happens to us is avoidable. But so many of the choices we are making right now will lead to whether we're vibrant at eighty, whether or not we get on that plane to see our child do something bigger than we could have ever dreamed up for him. Watching him make greatness out of tragedy.

This goal we have—the reason you're reading this book—is about you *feeling* amazing. But may I suggest that it's also about something bigger?

It's also about legacy. What kind of legacy are you going to leave? It's about what you did with your life. It's about whether you stretched yourself, learned the lessons, forged them into something that made your life and your family's lives better—or whether you just accepted the Law of Entropy as you slid downhill.

Remember, there's an opposite to the Law of Entropy—which is that the whole planet is upleveling in frequency. So momentum is on your side, and you can reverse the trajectory too! Technology and advances are making things possible that you should open your mind to. (I have a battery-powered car with no engine or transmission, and I can drive it from LA to New York City for free. Could you have imagined this just ten years ago?)

What will people say at your funeral and for years in the future about the way you lived and how that mattered to them?

The biggest thing I want you to get out of this chapter is to commit to checking in with yourself daily, many times, without judgment but just for the awareness of it:

"Is this [thought, action, statement] helping or hurting my vibration? How about others'? Is what I'm doing or saying right now helping or hurting my ViQ and others'?"

You're going to have the language of it, having read this. Whether you use this to change the way you walk on this earth is up to you. I'm here to support you. I'm visualizing you checking in every day, asking yourself:

"Is this helping or hurting my vibration?"

"Am I vibing with this person or not? Why? If I'm experiencing some low-vibration emotions or thoughts, is it me—or it is dissonant frequencies?"

"What can I do to upshift, get out of it, metabolize it, even use this lousy thing that happened to me as a catalyst to light up something good in my life?"

What I'm going to teach you in this chapter is very powerful. It's made as big a difference in my life as drinking gallons of green juice or smoothies every week has.

And I'm ecstatic to share it with you!

Let's go through an exercise to Metabolize/Reframe/Release a negative event, circumstance, or feeling. First we'll learn how significant, really, a "feeling" is. How long do you think the average emotion lasts? When you learn the answer to this question, you may wonder why your emotions have ruled you your whole life! Drumroll, please . . .

::::: THE NINETY-SECOND EMOTION :::::

That's right—research shows that the average emotion lasts just ninety seconds.

That's a fascinating fact that may be very helpful in your desire to have your life emphasize the positives, minimizing the negatives. Just knowing it may help you with metabolizing emotions if you remind yourself often, "This is just a feeling. It will go away." This has been important self-talk in my own lifelong fight with anxiety.

You can verify the truth of this if you think about what happens to you when you're discouraged and then you open a piece of mail or get a phone call with wonderful news—you're a new grandmother; you got the job of your dreams; someone you love and haven't seen in years is coming to town for a visit.

Have you ever had a difficult week, and then a friend sends you a really funny YouTube video that makes you laugh, not just once but over and over again every time you think of it—and especially when you share it with coworkers, and the whole office laughs about it all day?

And it completely changes your frequency, not just a mood or a "feeling" but perhaps even your productivity. Your views of events and people lift, and many other quick, energetic shifts take place that may affect you in a dozen different ways, all from laughing and sharing the laugh with others. You are very literally changing energetic trajectory, for both yourself and others.

Emotions can change quickly—and by that same logic, you can learn to manage the negatives to prevent an angry person or random event from taking your positive vibe from you.

Anxiety—or any other emotion—is nothing more than a wavelength, an energy, a set of frequencies. We tend to ascribe far too great a meaning to our every feeling—and for many people, those impulses, or energy bits, or feelings, rule and control their behavior, their mood, and even their outlook on life. Since 25 percent of Americans report feeling anxiety on a regular basis—some to a crippling extent that negatively impacts their quality of life—it's helpful to understand where emotion comes from.

Depression and anxiety, as chronic conditions, are often mistakenly seen as being related to a stressful situation. While a stressful situation can tip you over, from effectively handling your stress load into a zone you might define as no longer coping well, that situation is not, in fact, what you're anxious about, if you indeed have an anxiety disorder.

It's simply a trigger.

Entering his first term, President Franklin Delano Roosevelt said, "The only thing we have to fear is fear itself." This is a profound statement in the modern age, when severe anxiety is reported at a much higher rate than ever before. I'm far more afraid of anxiety—which at times has been excessive and, in fact, my greatest kryptonite in life—than I am of the actual something that might happen to me or my children or my business.

Anxiety, for me, is fairly easily controlled if I don't eat a significant amount of processed sugar, especially corn syrup; if I avoid drinking any alcohol besides that from the cleanest sources, and not too much or too often; and if I have challenges and "stress" in my life, but not so many that I'm emotionally tipped over by them.

In other words: don't eat sugar or processed foods, don't overdo alcohol, and do manage stress.

Sounds easy enough. But as with many things, I keep relearning these life lessons!

Rampant depression and anxiety disorders may stem from having more chemicals in our tissues than the body was ever intended to harbor, combined with the neurological system being maxed and unable to cope. With dozens of chemical plastics and chlorine and fluoride and other hormone disruptors in our environment, many if not most of us have an imbalanced endocrine (hormone) system. This is key in our feelings and our sense of well-being.

The anxiety epidemic may also be related to the many interruptions of our thoughts, our work, and our social time together that the electronic age has created—not to mention the breakneck pace of business, as so much of business has moved online with a proliferation of tools and software we're all supposed to know. More and more work output is required of any given employee at a company as more organizational and productivity tools roll out.

Simultaneously, we have less face time at the office and we work in isolated environments, many of us without the old-school meetings and collaborative work. Instead, most of us accomplish the majority of our work alone by typing and manipulating bits of digital data.

It's a social experiment the world has never experienced before.

So, aside from a chronic disorder such as clinical depression, generalized anxiety disorder, or panic disorder, we all deal with negative events and the inevitable resulting negative emotions.

::::: THE POWER OF NEUTRAL :::::

In order to be the director in the show that is your own life, it's necessary to stop being one of the characters and step back to get some perspective. Getting to a neutral space when negative intensity hits can be very powerful, in much the same way that, when driving a standard-transmission car, you step on the clutch before changing gears. (That reaction works so much better than just slamming on the brakes, screeching and jerking, doesn't it?)

It's not generally possible to go instantly from the fear and anger response triggered by someone screaming in your face, for instance, to imagining yourself floating in a pillowy cloud surrounded by sunshine, breezes, and love. There is a deliberate sequence of events, however, that can help you move through a stressful situation with grace and ease.

Many of the things we say or do in a moment of crisis have terrible long-term consequences. So the ability to assess, metabolize, sort, and move forward with clarity can be one of the most important things you ever learn.

Consider something you said once—early in your marriage, or to your young child, or to a coworker or close friend—that makes you wince just to think about. Perhaps, if you're like most of us, you've said or done something you deeply regret, the effect of which cannot be erased.

What would it be worth to you to be able to go back and retract a few things you've said or done over the years? A lot, right?

That's how important it is to learn to quickly assess, break down, make meaning of, make decisions about, and let go of a traumatic event.

As we get older, most of us learn to temper our speech. But even then, we make choices in a crisis that can literally cost lives, or relationships, or someone's health. Consider the swirling stories in the media about an innocent man with his hands in the air being shot by police because of multiple points of view of what was really going on at the scene, where everyone involved had to make split-second decisions.

Shifting into neutral so you can evaluate clearly, buy yourself a critical bit of time, and give yourself the space to decide which direction to go is terribly important. Because in a crisis, or a moment of anger or fear, in our paralysis we believe that we have only one course of action. And this can be tragic, because it is virtually never the case.

The ninety-second Metabolize/Reframe/Release method I developed, after a childhood and early adulthood of great trauma, has helped me in three very important ways, which I believe can have great power for you as well. I would never have been able to accomplish so much in my first fifty years had I not figured this out. Because the original coping mechanisms most of us develop in our early years are not very healthy or helpful.

The first great benefit to me of this technique is that it helps me to clear the energies of a flood of adrenaline, cortisol, and other stress hormones, and to gather myself to access my more intuitive perceptions and emotions. This allows me to make better decisions, even in a crisis.

I have often said, "People show who they are in extremity." Watch people in incredibly stressful situations, what they do and say. They prove their character when what they do is moral, selfless, or loving when it's difficult to be so.

Think of the person who takes the high road in divorce, refraining from slandering the other parent to the children, even though the other parent was unfaithful. Think of a person at the scene of a devastating accident who risks his own life to save others who are drowning or burning. Think of a politician who tells the truth despite the potential effect on her career.

Second, this ninety-second habit I will share with you helps me avoid living in a chronically stressed, anxious, and ultimately unhappy state. It's the rare person who almost never experiences traffic jams, unpleasant people, health challenges, children who make poor choices, and other stressors in their world. It's not the stressful events themselves that differentiate between consequences of health or illness; studies show us that it's primarily your perception of and reaction to those events that shapes your salvation or your demise.

Third, the ninety-second Metabolize/Reframe/Release method has helped me put negative events quickly and permanently in my rearview mirror, extracting only the "juice" of the learning opportunity available there and peacefully waving goodbye to the bad juju.

Researchers at the HeartMath Institute and elsewhere have studied how people who do not metabolize and make meaning of their life's challenges are those who suffer the worst outcomes of extreme life stressors such as losing a spouse or child, divorcing, moving far away, or being in a natural disaster.

For instance, some people who lose a child in an accident get therapy, process their grief, support others going through it, and share their positive memories and what they learned from going through their trial. Others who experienced the same thing spiral into substance or food addictions as an escape from the pain; their marriages break up, and life is never the same and never recovers. The Law of Attraction explains how as we move up or down in our frequencies, we attract more positives or more negatives, increasing the momentum of movement in either direction. (While this book leans toward Einstein's physics, I'll cite Newton here: Bodies in motion tend to stay in motion. Bodies at rest tend to stay at rest.)

Unchecked anger, depression, resentment, anxiety, and stress have the effect on your emotional and physical health of battery acid dripping on you twenty-four hours a day. They may have a worse effect than eating hot dogs, potato chips, and soda for lunch daily!

A number of decade-long studies show that chronic emotional stress is more predictive of death from cancer and heart disease than smoking is! In fact, you're 40 percent more likely to die of one of those diseases if you're chronically in these low-vibration states than if you're an individual who moves past challenges with grace and equanimity. The feeling of fear or anger is triggered by an event and is explained by a chain of biochemical responses in the sympathetic nervous system. It's a beautiful system that, since the dawn of man, means that if a ferocious lion is suddenly chasing you, your immune function shuts down to devote all of your faculties to what is most immediate. Your body knows it must react quickly, run, and defend. Your bowels may even evacuate, in the rush of stress hormones, as a lion lunges at you and your entire body goes into fight-or-flight mode.

In the modern age, we don't have lions chasing us—but the chronic overload of information and deadlines for professionals; the intensity of raising Millennials in a world of drugs, porn, materialism, and pressure to succeed; massive traffic in every major city; and many other stressors have many of us feeling that battery-acid drip of chronic stress.

Children let go of negative emotions quickly and easily, which can be astonishing to watch as an adult. We wonder what they have that we don't. When did we lose that ability to release negatives promptly?

The difference is that we've adopted patterns of replaying negative events and feelings in our minds and with our words, telling other people about them, processing them, "baking" them into a hard-coded reality.

If a small child tells you about falling and skinning her knee, it's for comfort or for a solution to it. If we retell a negative event, we're incubating and imprinting negatives in all our energies, without realizing the self-sabotage incurred; we're learning to perpetuate negativity as a pattern.

Deepak Chopra teaches that most of our thoughts are negative—thousands of them every day, many of them toward ourselves—and an astonishing 95 percent of these negative thoughts are just on "replay": we think the same gloomy thoughts every hour, every day, every year.

Energies can heal—and the flip side of that is that energies can kill. What's exciting is that becoming aware of how most of our negative thoughts are just replaying on a loop is the beginning of turning that around!

Go back to the introduction and take a look at those two charts again, of the 200 seconds of ECG results showing the heart frequencies of a person feeling anger versus a person feeling deep gratitude. Notice that they literally *look like* how anger and gratitude feel!

The parasympathetic nervous system is a counterbalancing system that optimizes when you are relaxed: reading a book about something positive, sitting outside in the sunshine taking deep breaths, or enjoying candlelight and a glass of wine or cup of tea in a beautiful setting with someone you love.

Both parts of the nervous system have important functions. But if your negative emotions are lasting more than ninety seconds on average, you may want to do two things. First, try examining whether you are prolonging those feelings by talking about them excessively or dwelling on them more than is useful.

And, second, you may want to practice the ninety-second Metabolize/Reframe/Release technique of asking yourself questions to get clarity about where the emotion came from, and then dissipating it. The result will be that you sidestep the self-poisoning of tension and stress that can affect your vibration and, therefore, your health over time.

It has been very helpful for me, as I'm feeling an uncomfortable emotion, to remind myself, "This is nothing more nor less than a feeling. It's going to go away soon, and it's here to teach me something. What would that be?"

I am able to calm myself down this way, being very rational and purposeful about resolving a feeling, much as I resolve any other challenge in my path, and reminding myself that I can minimize the amount of time I spend in this uncomfortable, sick feeling.

Another thing I remind myself is that it isn't the awful thing someone said to me that is the poison, it's my reaction to it. And I can choose a different reaction.

I don't smother or deny the emotion. I spend a moment in the Metabolize/Reframe/Release process we're about to dive into to find the purpose or lesson in what I'm feeling, use it as fuel for my own growth and upleveling, and release it from the job it's done so well, with gratitude for the lesson once I'm finished with it.

Big tragedies in our lives aren't resolved in ninety seconds, of course. If you were sexually abused for ten years in your childhood by a person who was supposed to protect you, or if your house burned down along with everything you own, you won't be able to do the work of unpacking that and putting it to rest in mere minutes.

There are many layers to such traumatic events, and they deserve the time you take to explore them with a professional therapist or coach and, if you're blessed to have such a person, with someone you love and trust absolutely. However, once the key awarenesses are clear and you know the path forward, you can check in with yourself anytime your issues related to that trauma are triggered in the daily events of life, and those feelings can be useful and then released in peace in a very short time.

You'll want to metabolize your emotions and give what you've learned to the universe for the sake of the good karma that's going to flow your way if you stay in the positive energetics rather than the negative ones.

:::: RESOLVE ANY NEGATIVE EMOTION :::: IN NINETY SECONDS OR LESS!

Using a couple of stories from my own life, I'm going to walk you slowly through a process in which someone enters your energy field and does something awful that you don't deserve, and before you're done, you're wishing him well, releasing all negative emotion, and leaving it behind—and you're happier than you were before it all happened.

I'm not kidding.

It's not for everyone. As I said a few pages back, if you want to be a victim, if you want to stay in whatever stuck place you're in because it serves you in some way, then this is not for you. If you spend a lot of your time talking about negative stories, this may rob you of some of your conversation. That could be a drag.

But if you want a high-vibration life, every day, every month, every year? Even while bad juju happens all over the globe and in your own world? Then you absolutely must master this.

And guess what? Even though we're going to go through it slowly, you can do all of this, when you get good at it, in ninety seconds or less! And you can do it anytime, anywhere, without anyone even knowing.

Let's start with *Metabolizing*. If you don't digest the negative emotion, it will keep festering, bubbling up, and resurfacing, affecting many parts of your life. Just like undigested food in your gut, it will eventually make you sick.

To metabolize an emotion, ask yourself the following two questions—and do not go on to the second question until you clearly know the answer to the first. You'll eventually become very quick at this, so that you can complete the entire process in just seconds:

Q1: Why I am feeling angry [or uncomfortable, frustrated, anxious, discouraged]—what is really bothering me, beneath the surface emotion?

Make a one- or two-sentence statement to yourself. Often the clarity alone, after answering this first question, moves stuck energies forward significantly.

Example: "I'm unable to focus because I keep thinking about what my boss, Connie, said. I can't tell if she's unhappy with my work, and I didn't have the presence of mind to ask her when I was in her office."

Example: "I feel hurt and misunderstood because I sense my children are siding with my ex-husband, and they don't seem to want to hear my position on why I said what I did."

Q2: Now that I know what's really eating at me, what actions could I take to solve it?

Example: "I could send Connie an e-mail. The timing is important, because I want to write it when I'm not assuming anything. Maybe I shouldn't write an e-mail—then I still don't know what she's thinking, and I want to see her body language. I'll stop into her office after lunch. I'll gather my thoughts right now and think how to ask it. I'll be really warm and encourage her to be forthright with me. I'll preempt any unhappiness she has about my work by telling her really clearly how important it is to me to do a good job, that I welcome her feedback, and that I have a sense she may not be completely happy with my work."

Example: "Maybe I need to sit with this and not try to solve it with the kids right now. They're dug in, they're reactive, and they're expecting me to criticize their dad because I've done so in the past. I could let the situation lie until I've expressed support and love for each one of the kids before bringing it up again—stay in the love zone, not the reaction zone. Maybe by then I will have realized that this isn't even important. If I give this three days and just love the kids up, maybe this will blow over and I won't care about it. And if it still feels substantial, I can always bring it up when their feelings settle down."

After asking yourself these first two questions to metabolize what's *really* going on, you may have a plan in mind that resolves the emotion and has the additional benefit of movement toward solving a problem. Often, when I ask myself questions to get to the bottom of why I'm stuck in a low-vibe state, I find that I am worried about something. I then schedule a time to worry! That's right: I table it, because I know it needs attention that I can't give it right now.

For instance, if I'm struggling with getting my teenage son to help around the house without our relationship becoming contentious, and that dynamic is causing me anxiety as I'm working, I'll schedule myself to think about it during a fifteen-minute drive to a meeting that afternoon, and then I'll schedule myself to chat with my son that night.

Other times, though, checking in with myself ("Why am I feeling _____?") helps me get clear within mere seconds about why I'm not optimizing my ViQ and what needs to happen in order to get back in sync with my purposes. Many times, all I need is simply awareness and choosing a shift, using any of the practices that raise vibration described in this book and/or the ninety-second process that follows.

The ability to live in the grounded frequencies starts with awareness of the principles you're discovering in this book and making a commitment to choosing a high-vibration life. It truly must start with choice.

The Six-Question Process in Action, Adding Reframe and Release

Now let's take a fast-action issue involving anger as an example. Let's say you turn out of a parking lot and don't see a car coming up fast until the driver has to slam on his brakes and swerve. He then speeds around you in the lane beside yours and makes an obscene gesture. Let's try the exercise now, only let's take it a few steps further.

Q1: Why I am feeling angry [or uncomfortable, frustrated, anxious, discouraged]—what is really bothering me, beneath the surface emotion?

Example: "I really feel guilty that I almost caused an accident and I am feeling remorseful about my mistake. But I also think he's overreacting, and that's a really vulgar gesture I don't appreciate. He's made driving mistakes too! So now I feel angry. And I feel a bit scared. I don't know if he's a road-rage kind of guy."

Q2: Now that I know what's really eating at me, what actions could I take to solve it?

Example: "I could flip him off and be really aggressive, slamming on my brakes or stepping on the gas to get away from him. Then he'd know how angry I am, and I'd 'pay him back.'"

Now we're moving on to the *Reframe*, where you'll ask yourself questions to completely change your mindset and point of view, which is fantastically helpful for getting out of stuck vibrations. In a stressful situation, for most people unpracticed in these techniques, your ego takes over and you're operating from what I, as a therapist, call "lizard brain" (the limbic system), which is quick to anger and is rarely helpful in human interactions—unless you're in danger. (And usually when we go to lizard brain, we actually aren't in danger!)

By asking yourself the following questions, you're moving your thought processes from the limbic brain to the frontal lobe, where you're far more likely to be consequence-oriented, operating with a longer-range view, and compassionate. (In short, the frontal lobe of your brain will help you move into higher vibrations.)

Q3: If I felt and did the opposite of what my first instinct was, or did something very different, what would I do?
Example: "I'd smile and wave, as if he's a very dear friend I haven't seen in a while."

Q4: How would it feel to do that—and which will I choose?
Whatever you choose, I'm not here to disapprove. I'm suggesting that a reframe might just take a burden off your shoulders. You can't reframe anything until you know precisely what it is (metabolize). And reframing is another exciting step toward making a conscious choice, toward our end goal of being able to scatter the ashes of the negative situation in the wind, keeping only the learning opportunity (release) and moving forward in the higher frequencies.

Make your choice whether to go with your instinct from the first moment you felt the low vibrations or the more thoughtful and precise *opposite* or *very different* approach. (Some would call this "the high road.") To encourage you to at least try the latter, remember that one comes from your limbic or reptilian brain, where teenagers usually live, and the other comes from your prefrontal cortex, where sophisticated and thoughtful adults living purposeful lives live.

Whichever you chose, make sure you take a moment, when the intensity of the negative situation has dissipated, and evaluate. Ask your two last questions. Once the intensity passes (remember, nothing intense lasts, whether good or bad), we're ready to *Release* this experience.

Shake off the negative energetics of how it all started by asking yourself these final questions. Then you can let go of the "waste products" of your metabolizing bad vibrations, keeping only the learning opportunity:

Q5: How did that feel, what were the consequences, and did it raise or lower my ViQ?

Example: "When I flipped the guy off in response, and he rolled his window down and escalated the obscenities, I felt my blood pressure go up and I spent the better part of an hour reliving it in my mind, thinking about what I should have said back, and feeling angry. I couldn't focus at work. Then later I told Sweetie about it and felt the rage all over again (and wrecked her vibe after a long day at work). This event defined and ruined my day."

Example: "When I smiled and waved, I had to try not to laugh. It felt pretty grounded to make a decision that wasn't from my limbic brain! I think he wanted a reaction out of me, to know that he'd gotten under my skin. I wish him peace and all the best. This might have actually made him think a bit about his own road rage. I'd be really embarrassed if I gave somebody the bird, and that person was kind to me in response. I'm kind of proud of myself, because I've never kept my cool in that situation before. I feel like today I'm doing my part to uplevel my whole town's collective frequency! Pay-it-forward stuff. Maybe that guy will treat someone who makes a driving mistake with compassion later. Can't wait to tell Sweetie when she gets home."

Q6: What can I learn from this for the future?

I will let you sit for a moment with the power that asking yourself a few questions, before making a limbic-brain decision, can have in your life, especially as you practice doing the opposite and finding out which you prefer.

You just turned a doorknob and you're seeing the sunshine, possibly for the first time in your life. I hope the freedom from being trapped in your own bad vibes feels like magic, smells like fresh air, and tastes like exhilaration.

The reason I used this example of someone flipping you off in traffic is that it's a common experience and we've all had it. I want to recommend that you try this approach in that kind of situation.

See what you learn from it that is applicable to other daily situations in your life. This is similar to the process that Zen Buddhist masters and other deeply spiritual human beings from disciplines around the globe go through—who, with years of practice, learn to live in a peaceful state virtually all of the time.

You can find these six questions on your Resources page and print them out. Have a copy at work and another at home until you've internalized them, to help this short process become a habit that just might change your life for the better.

At an ashram where I did research in Texas, I met a man who was there for a spiritual retreat to address his anger problems. I asked him where he experienced the anger, expecting to hear him mention his spouse or his children, but his answer surprised me: "I experience road rage almost every day." For him, keeping the list of questions in the car probably makes the most sense! Where should you keep your list of questions?

Long before road rage, the great stoic Marcus Aurelius told us to prepare for the fact that the day will bring negatives, and that we have a choice in how we will handle them:

> When you first rise in the morning, tell yourself: I will encounter busybodies, ingrates, egomaniacs, liars, the jealous, and cranks. They are all stricken with these afflictions because they don't know the difference between good and evil. Because I have understood the beauty of good and the ugliness of evil, I know that these wrong-doers are still akin to me . . . and that none can do me harm or implicate me in ugliness—nor can I be angry at my relatives or hate them. For we are made for cooperation.
>
> *Meditations 2.1*

Now Let's Look at an Example

Long ago, I "reframed" a travel day, from previously considering it a waste of time to now seeing it as a day of people-watching and unique productivity. I get so much done and have had some of my very best ideas on flights.

This particular time, I got on a plane, and the guy sitting next to me was clicking his pen. Over and over. Nonstop, thousands of times. This went on for ten or fifteen minutes, to the point where I realized—this was just what he did. This would be my reality for the next three hours.

I felt the sound waves of the clicking pen interrupting the flow of the work I was trying to do. I couldn't think clearly. I was, very frankly, annoyed and distracted.

The first thing I did was *Metabolize* what was going on. If you eat a banana, it doesn't sit in your stomach as a banana, right? You metabolize it, and it goes through many processes and moves through different parts of your thirty feet of gastrointestinal tract, and eventually it becomes energy in cells, or ATP. Emotions can be the same way, and I welcome a challenge to take some input and metabolize it for my own good.

So I began to metabolize this entire situation, breaking it down. I asked myself questions, and they started very, very simply.

The first one is always: *What am I feeling right now—why am I uncomfortable or unhappy?*

["Well, I'm annoyed. I'm inconvenienced. I wanted to concentrate and get into a flow with my work, and instead I'm thinking about this dumb guy and his obsessive-compulsive disorder."]

Next question: *Could I solve this problem? If so, how?*

["Well, yes, I could ask him to stop. Very nicely. If that doesn't work, I could ask the flight attendant to reseat me. Or get her to ask him to stop. Things would get pretty uncomfortable, and people around us would probably choose sides. I could even go to the micro-phone, grab it, and ask if there's a psychiatrist on the plane, because a mentally ill gentleman is next to me and I need an intervention. . . . Okay, I'm getting a bit carried away. The point is, yes, I could solve this problem, rather than just being annoyed. So I can ask him to stop. He probably will stop."]

Now I moved on to the *Reframe*: *What else could I do, how else can I see this, that is for my own growth and learning, that doesn't involve so much negative vibration and isn't all about my ego?* (Note that there are *always* other legitimate points of view. We cannot see them when we are in limbic brain.) What would be the opposite of asking him to stop, and what might that feel like? Reframing is purposefully adopting a completely different point of view, which is powerful in shifting mood, mindset, and, literally, the part of the brain from which you think and make decisions.

["Well, I could do a little experiment. I could take a few minutes and take slow, deep breaths and tell myself a story about what this man has been through to acquire such nervous habits. Clearly, he has anxiety. I wonder if he has Asperger's and he doesn't read social cues well enough to understand that people don't like constant pen-clicking right next to them. That would be really stressful and scary and sad. I bet that's hard for him. His mom isn't in his life anymore, and Dad has had a string of subsequent wives, and the man has never been a priority. I bet he has a cat who just died. Wow, some people would become alcoholic over all that! Clicking a pen is a small thing that doesn't really hurt anyone. Geez. There are people who hurt others when they're hurting; all he's doing is clicking a pen. I feel sad for him, and I love him. I want the best for him. I hope that he gets to a happier place."]

Let me tell you what happened next, which is *Release*. I settled into an energetic space of pure Zen. I felt at peace in my cramped seat, having fully immersed myself in the high-vibration emotions of compassion and love—which were a challenge to feel, but *I absolutely can do it at will, and by choice*—and I felt free to be creative, writing in my notebook. I felt 100 percent at peace with the pen-clicking—I'd released the negative emotion, which is quite easy after finding something positive in the situation.

It simply did not bother me anymore. Not for one second. I cranked out a bunch of work that was meaningful to me, I was "in the zone," I enjoyed the flight as I always do, and I reinforced an important lesson.

This is just an example. Worse things happen to you in any given month than having to sit next to someone with an annoying, noisy habit on a plane.

However, situations like this are common. Over time, small things that we cannot let go of and invest negative energy in become cancer. They become a hard heart. They become an inability to engage authentically, in a vulnerable way, with other human beings because we judge them harshly and quickly.

I've given you a printable version of this exact list of questions I ask myself in order to metabolize an emotion by identifying it, breaking it down so I fully understand it, reframing it to make a good decision and to find the opportunity in it, and then letting all of it go except for the golden nugget of learning that serves me. (Grab and print this list from your Resources page.)

I highly recommend that you check in with yourself before you react, breaking down and metabolizing the situation and the emotion, asking yourself how you might see it differently and deal with it differently than Neanderthal man would, and then trying to do the opposite—or at least something very different than your first response.

Something compassionate. Something so unexpectedly merciful that it changes your heart. That completely changes the charge between you and a stranger, or between you and a friend. This works with anyone and anything.

You never know what burden someone is carrying, so it's good to follow Plato's wise counsel.

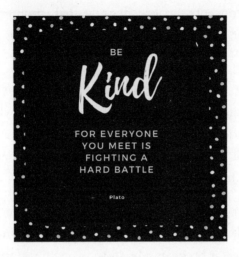

::::: ARE LOW-VIBE EMOTIONS BAD? :::::

When Pen-Clicker Guy gets on the plane next to you, do you have *choices*? What are they? Empower yourself that you *could* do the low-vibe thing. Fear, anger, and anxiety, after all, do have a purpose, and they are important.

They tell you when there's danger. They tell you that action is needed.

If Handgun Guy somehow got on the plane instead of Pen-Clicker Guy, and stuck his weapon in your ribs and threatened you, fear and anger would be very important emotions in helping you solve the problem, right? Negative emotions can be useful, especially to quickly move us to a better place.

The problem arises, affecting your health and your ability to be happy, when one of three things happens with those low-vibe feelings:

1. You don't metabolize and release that emotion quickly. So it ends up literally trapped in the proteins of your body. You've read enough of this book by now to understand that "every-

thing in life is vibration." (Here's a mini-quiz: Who said that? Ten points if you said Albert Einstein!) So it doesn't seem a foreign concept anymore, does it—that emotion is part of the "matter" or physical substances in your body? All of it is energy.

2. Another problem with low-vibe emotions—which, let's face it, are just part of the human experience—is when anger, fear, or anxiety isn't serving. It's not helping you accomplish anything or move you to action—it's just paralyzing you and eating you from the inside, like battery acid.

3. The third problem is that while those negative emotions may occasionally serve a purpose, you may be experiencing them far too much: it becomes a brain-wavelength pattern when it's chronic. And we've already established that anger as a steady diet is as bad for you as a steady diet of french fries—maybe worse!

So one of the very best things you can do as you move toward your high-vibration life is to get really serious about Metabolizing/Reframing/Releasing negative emotions.

If you're feeling negative emotions several times a day or more, here are three good questions to ask yourself:

- Do I feel anger, fear, or anxiety more than I'd like to?
- Have I lost track of when these emotions serve and when they don't?
- Am I willing to undergo a short process and commit to breaking these vibes down so that I can feel them less frequently and let go of them more quickly?

If you said yes to any of those questions, mastering this exercise is going to be a game changer for you! And, as with all good habits, you won't master it by doing it just once or twice.

Let's go back to when Pen-Clicker Guy sits next to you on the airplane. And you have begun to become very conscious of the fact that you have choices. Give yourself permission to lash out, say something snarky, engage the flight attendant, commandeer the cockpit microphone. . . .

I'm being ridiculous. But you and I both know that many times we've seen people go up in the anger elevator to the 114th floor over small things, ending up in a bizarre, overwrought situation due to completely uncontrolled Neanderthal impulses.

If you have ever gone to the 114th floor in the anger elevator in six seconds, let me ask you:

How did it feel? What happened to your vibration? Was it worth it?

What if you missed an opportunity for personal growth? How can you reframe and be in a completely different happiness frequency after just a few minutes?

I've described for you my *actual* experience with Pen-Clicker Guy. Does the result I experienced sound more appealing to you than what happens—how you feel, what it does to your vibe and others'—when you're screaming into a microphone at 150 passengers, demanding that a psychiatrist present herself immediately?

Or just sitting there, silently seething, still annoyed every time you think about Pen-Clicker Guy later?

Chronic anger, whether expressed or suppressed, is truly toxic. (Ditto depression, self-criticism, anxiety, worry, jealousy, and any other of the negative vibes I've missed!) In fact, a very old study showed that women who have passive personalities and "stuff" their feelings get breast cancer at significantly higher rates. This is evidence that in addition to the magnetics of your behavior, the energies of your emotion can make you sick, whereas dealing with them and releasing them peacefully leads to health.

:::: HOW YOU COMMUNICATE :::: NEGATIVES MATTERS

Crucial Conversations is one of my favorite books about communication. Its four PhD authors (Patterson et. al.) researched who the employees were in large companies whom others trusted and went to with their problems. They weren't always management employees, though sometimes they were. Someone didn't have to be in a position of leadership for other employees to point to them as the one they enlisted to listen and help solve major problems. What the authors discovered is that most of us take one of two roads in our communication:

Silence or violence.

Now, violence is well understood. Swearing, scolding, shaming, belittling, shouting—these are behaviors we've all seen from bullies, even bullies in the workplace. These energies are aggressive and obvious. But the revolutionary discovery in these researchers' work is that the "silent treatment" types, the passive-aggressives, do every bit as much harm.

They may feel they're nicer or in some way superior, but, in fact, giving someone the "silent treatment"—stonewalling, telling the person you'll do as they asked and then sabotaging the plan, speaking ill of someone behind their back with words you'd never say to their face—is at least as harmful to a relationship, or a work project, as the damage that "violence" folks cause.

And those you trust, in your personal or professional life, are those who take the middle path. It's very narrow, and very few traverse it. But the *Crucial Conversations* researchers discovered that those who do are highly trusted and much loved. They aren't necessarily the "nicest" in the company, but they are willing to have the difficult conversations. They say what needs to be said. They confront the elephant in the room.

But they do it with respect, with a genuine desire to make everyone in the situation whole, and with clear, straightforward words. They may "call you out"—they may even fire you. But—and this is what most people go their entire lives not realizing—these people often actually strengthen their relationships with others by telling them hard things.

This may be counterintuitive to a person who avoids conflict. Those who gain the most respect from others navigate conflict with the courage to be clear and direct as well as kind and compassionate. Those sets of qualities are not mutually exclusive, and few people know this.

If you're in an intimate relationship with someone who is all of those things—clear, direct, unflinching about facing and resolving conflict, but also compassionate and kind—do whatever you must to keep that person in your life. He or she is a unicorn! You have every possibility of enjoying a high-vibration relationship with this person, because your partner is capable of it. (Are you?)

You'll want to evaluate whether you resort to silence or violence or both, and then ask yourself whether this is serving you and your relationships. (Try to avoid assigning blame outside yourself, such as: "Well, I would be direct and clear if he weren't always [negative behavior trait].")

Is it a revelation to you that people actually love working with someone who communicates his frustrations or dissatisfactions—judiciously, of course, but openly, honestly, on occasion even bluntly—but always with an energy of kindness, love, and respect, giving colleagues and friends an opportunity to clear the air?

If that is indeed a revelation to you, there's great news here:

You're on your way to a breakthrough in not only your ViQ but also in a whole world of amazing interactions with other people, from this day forward!

:::: HIGH-VIBE AND LOW-VIBE EMOTIONS ::::

Positive Energetic States

I hope you'll internalize the idea that spending more time, more moments of your life, turning your attention to the high-vibe emotions can have a huge impact on your quality of life and even your disease risk. Whether or not an underlying chemical issue underpins your low-vibration depression or anxiety pattern, whether or not you take a chemical drug for it, shifting mindset and gaining control over your emotions *must be part of the long-term solution.*

As the speed of life increases, technology accelerates, we encounter toxins everywhere in the environment, and the entire world becomes more competitive—consequently, we find degrading brain patterns associated with these phenomena. Some of us are handling rapidly changing realities and increasing stresses better than others.

None of us can afford for circumstances to dictate our ViQ! We need to keep our ability to focus, our trend toward concentrating on the positives, and our problem-solving capability intact!

After all, each of us encounters both positive and negative circumstances every day, in each of our unique situations. Whichever of them gets most of our focus—in the minutes of thought, the depth of emotion, and the energies we attach to the events of our lives in conversations with others—heavily influences our electrical energetics and those of other people who enter our field.

I'm about to share with you words that each evoke a state of high vibration that you will have your own personal, unique reaction to—but they are words with universally positive associations that take disciplined practice to pull into your thought patterns daily.

Rate how often you consciously or unconsciously experience the following positive states of mind:

1 = almost never
2 = occasionally
3 = fairly often
4 = very often
5 = often or daily

Scores of 4 or 5 are wonderful, so congratulate yourself on those! Any words that you give a score of 1 to 3 are ones you should print on a 3x5 card to put on your mirror or bring to your meditation practice, to practice visualizing and creating these states in your mind. As you practice, your other energies, such as actions and words, will follow.

Folks who can truthfully circle 4 or 5 on all of these states are those with Optimal ViQ. If that describes you, take your strategies out into the world to save everyone else from all the low frequencies!

How much do I experience these states daily?		
Gratitude	1 2 3 4 5	Peace	1 2 3 4 5
Optimism	1 2 3 4 5	Calm	1 2 3 4 5
Empathy	1 2 3 4 5	Fulfillment	1 2 3 4 5
Love	1 2 3 4 5	Purpose	1 2 3 4 5
Joy	1 2 3 4 5	Flow	1 2 3 4 5
Fun	1 2 3 4 5	Abundance	1 2 3 4 5

I've made you a PDF you can print with each of these one-word ViQ-raising emotions on it, as well as the negative emotion chart on page 66. (Find it on your Resources page.) Circle any positive emotion you're not experiencing enough of and post it where you can see it every day.

That's your reminder to infuse the thought, the associated energies, and the upvibing into your consciousness daily. As you do the 10-Minute, Five-in-One Yoga Flow, which I explain in the next chapter, you can replace the meditation with simply saying the word you're working on upon each exhale as you breathe.

In some cases, an action must precede the emotion. You may have difficulty experiencing purpose or fun or fulfillment if you aren't actively doing anything. You might struggle to experience love or empathy unless you're in a relationship of some kind with another person. So this is the perfect illustration of how emotional states tend to change as actions change.

Negative Energetic States

Some emotions may serve a short-term purpose to alert us to danger or motivate us to action. But if they are experienced chronically and without resolution, they tax the sympathetic nervous system, impair the brain, alienate other people, keep us from being offered opportunities, and prevent high-quality relationships—leaving us vaguely or even acutely dissatisfied with life and wondering why.

Rate how often you consciously or unconsciously experience these negative states of mind:

1 = almost never
2 = occasionally
3 = fairly often
4 = very often
5 = often or daily

Scores of 3 to 5 indicate negative states you want to become mindful of; using tapping (see chapter 3) and/or the Metabolize/Reframe/Release method described earlier can dramatically decrease how much power these energies have on your ViQ. For any negative energetic state on which you rated yourself 1 or 2, congratulate yourself that you are doing well in avoiding these energy vampires!

How much do I experience these states daily?		
Resistance	1 2 3 4 5	Self-Doubt 1 2 3 4 5
Anxiety	1 2 3 4 5	Jealousy 1 2 3 4 5
Shame	1 2 3 4 5	Fear 1 2 3 4 5
Anger	1 2 3 4 5	Critical of Self 1 2 3 4 5
		or Others

It's important to evaluate, spending thirty to sixty seconds on each of these emotions, whether you're dwelling in any of these negatives. Most of us will discover that we have a tendency toward one or more of them, while others are not a problem for us. (Consider it a blessing if one or more of these is not holding you back!) Resistance to what is can result in feelings of being stuck. Resistance to accepting reality can also result in avoiding doing things you want to achieve, whether it be developing a skill more completely, finishing a project, or losing ten pounds.

Finding the balance between fixing issues in your life (active problem-solving) and releasing emotion about what cannot be changed (active acceptance) is one of the greatest keys to upvibing.

Take whichever of these words felt most like your own specific challenges into the Metabolize/Reframe/Release method you've learned, and consider trying out tapping, also called the Emotional Freedom Technique (EFT), in the next chapter, to make quicker work of resolving your negative emotions each time you experience them. Be sure to read the Meditation section coming up in the next chapter—and consider using your 3x5 cards, noting each negative state you experience often, to release that state as you meditate for a few minutes each day.

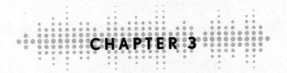

CHAPTER 3

Practices that Raise Vibration

THINGS THAT RAISE

• Doing Challenging & Meaningful
Mental or Physical Work

• Being Outdoors in Nice Weather & Sunshine

• Consciously Cultivating Gratitude & Peace

• Deep Breathing

• Being Around Self-Actualizing, Positive People

• Pets

• Mindfulness

• EFT/Tapping

• Mastery of Emotions

• Letting Go of What Doesn't Serve

• Sexual Energetics

One of the most important takeaways I hope you get from this book is that your every simple choice in the course of a day affects your energies. Let's go through some of them that are the most powerful and easy to implement. We'll start with the positives!

Challenging and Meaningful Mental or Physical Work

Having problems to solve, including complex projects, is good for the brain's long-term viability and, as it turns out, is also good for your sense of purpose and well-being. The same can be said for having work that makes a difference in the lives of others, which is highly gratifying in many ways.

And I have noticed that those who sell cars, write legal contracts, or manufacture physical products often describe loving their work because they feel it helps others. So you don't have to be a doctor, an inspirational speaker, or a therapist to experience the powerful vibrations of helping others every day while being paid.

We all need to feel that we have a reason to be on the planet, and the most common complaint of those who commit suicide is a feeling of meaninglessness. Even if your job is assembly-line work, doing it with others, doing it well, and doing it with goals and some kind of challenge to it is just plain good for you. This type of challenge is the perfect example of how "stress" in the sense of having tension in your life is actually a positive; the kind of stress that is bad for you and your vibe is chronic negatives in life that are not being resolved.

I often say that I've been blessed to have a career doing precisely what I want to do and chose to do. I'd been passionate for many years about teaching people to eat whole foods. In the beginning, I had no goal of earning a living this way. I just offered many free classes, with nothing for sale. I was simply showing the easy, delicious, cheap ways I'd learned to feed my family whole foods, get them off the processed-food train (ditching our diagnoses and drugs along the way), and lose a lot of weight.

I even traveled out of state to teach classes. My online following offered me spaces to teach and sponsors, and even after I wrote my first book, I'd often forget to take copies to sell to attendees. Or I'd forget to take small bills to make change, because I was so absorbed in preparing my demos and class materials. It was truly a mission, and financial benefit didn't even occur to me. As my website took more and more of my time, I felt called to quit my guaranteed-income university job and devote myself to it.

But karma rewards passion and integrity. Karma flows in the form of attraction to all the right things. I have a voice in my head when things don't seem to be flowing, and it goes like this:

"Trust karma. The universe is perfect. It all works out."

I would rather make less money doing something I can be excited about that has me jumping out of bed every morning because I want to dive into it. So at GreenSmoothieGirl.com, I taught what I knew and loved, regardless of whether I had a big marketing "play" for any content I spent my time on.

I required of myself that I work on my limiting beliefs. Those included fretting over the fact that I'm technically inept, I struggle with spreadsheets, and I never got that MBA I should probably have to run a business—I can name half a dozen pain points in my business at any given time.

All of the growth that had to happen came with time and with a lot of consistent effort. I have many more hurdles to jump and things to learn in my career. I've learned that I love the challenges, even though sometimes my ambitious plans take my breath away if I allow myself to tune in to the fear vibration.

I did find ways to make a living while doing precisely what I wanted to, and I offered nothing to my audience that I wasn't doing myself and wasn't convinced would make their lives better.

In short, I've been able to run a business teaching people to eat whole foods, which is what resuscitated my own health many years ago, very successfully and with integrity.

And the reason I want to share this with you is that my work is truly one of the greatest blessings of my life. I often say to my children, "Work is a blessing." I do not want them to think of it as a chore, something they count the minutes and hours until they can stop doing. Work can, and should, fuel your high-vibration life as much as anything can!

I get to do something meaningful that helps others, that challenges me, and that supports my family well. If you can't say the same, I hope you do whatever it takes to live your life in a bigger way in terms of what you do to pay the bills.

Get that certification, work those extra hours, do things that scare you, ask someone in your network for an introduction. It's okay to be scared—who isn't?—but it's not okay to not go for your dreams because you're scared. That's low-vibe living.

Living high-vibe isn't always hard. But living low-vibe is a bit easier in the day-to-day choices, because you eat whatever tastes good, you rarely get out of the chair—hence the fact that most people live in inertia, slumped in a chair, and die there.

We spend so much of our lives doing work; it's imperative that what we choose, professionally, be positive and joyful.

Keep in mind that my career has not been easy. Not by a long shot. Nor do I like everything in my day or everything about my job. I think a fantastic job is one you like or love 80 to 90 percent of, and you find ways to be at peace with the other 10 to 20 percent—and do it anyway, thanking God daily for the challenge.

I've had bad days, bad months, and even a bad entire year, when it comes to challenges or stress. I've had at least five people threaten to sue me along the way, without any legitimate reason beyond bad assumptions, greed, and competition. I've made mistakes that have cost me at least a million dollars in losses. I've worked with dishonest partners and employees who stole money from me.

I've sustained many other losses, have had to fire several employees over the course of eight years, and passionately invested a great deal of time and effort into things that didn't pan out.

I've failed, big, a number of times.

And still, I have what by anyone's standards can only be called a very successful business and a successful, amazing, adventurous, and now even debt-free life.

To achieve your dreams, you just have to win a bit more than you lose, learn to be calm and centered even in the storm, and write off your losses as quickly as you write off your negative emotions. Coming to peace with the fact that life includes some losses and putting my setbacks in my rearview mirror as quickly as possible, while keeping the key learnings, has been one of the most important things I've ever learned how to do.

Being Outside in Nice Weather: Sunshine, Oxygen, Interaction with Living Things

Being outside lets you fill your lungs with clean air and detoxify an important part of your body. And sunshine isn't just good for the soul; it's also critical in preventing cancer and building healthy bones. Sunshine has now been proven to recharge the human "battery."

The sun's rays have been demonized as being cancer-causing, and dermatologists told us for decades to stay out of the sun and slather on sunscreen. In fact, many still do. It's true that sunburns can lead to cancer—at least the most innocuous kinds, basal and squamous cell cancers, which are almost always easily treated. However, it's looking more likely that truly deadly skin cancer, melanoma, is not caused by sun damage.

Hundreds of studies have been published proving that vitamin D levels are the number one correlate to cancer risk of all kinds. That is, the closer people live to the equator, with more sun exposure, the higher their vitamin D levels and the lower their cancer incidence is. This has turned skin cancer assumptions and research upside down.

We all know we breathe too much stale, dirty air in exhaust-choked cities and inside office spaces, and that we need to get outside. But what else is in the sunshine, the clean air, and the great outdoors that can radically shift our sense of well-being in one hour outside?

Not only can you "bank" vitamin D against the sunless winter months, to a certain extent, but sunshine and oxygenating clean air increase endorphins and make you healthier and happier. What do you most like to do outside? My twenty-two-year-old daughter and I have a favorite hike near our home, from the Sundance resort up to a wonderful waterfall. My seventeen-year-old son and I love to ski together, which can sometimes get us some sun in the winter. Plus, we take our vacation in a warm place when it's the dead of winter here in Utah.

It's important to note that vitamin D on the surface of your skin takes time to absorb and assimilate, so, if possible, don't shower for a few hours after being outside in the sun for a while.

More and more evidence is emerging that commercial sunscreens are full of chemicals that lead, ironically, to cancer. The worst are the aerosol cans that have even more harmful chemicals. You can purchase physical or mineral (versus chemical) sunblocks online and at health food stores that are free of harmful chemicals and use titanium dioxide to block the sun's harmful rays. You can even buy a tinted version, such as from the company Green Screen. That way, the lotion doesn't make you look pasty white, which is usually the complaint about these sunscreens.

Being outside exposes you to harmonic vibrations that have the opposite effect on your health than those indoors, where all the electrical gadgets are plugged in. For most of us in urban environments, being outside requires planning, purposefully choosing to recharge in the clean air of a natural environment. Because I often work from home, I go outside for work calls anytime the weather is inviting.

Consciously Cultivating Gratitude and Peace

Often, when I find myself starting into a negative thought and emotion pattern, because of so much conditioning at a young age and a childhood of physical and emotional abuse and resulting PTSD, I interrupt those thoughts with a reflection on the things I'm grateful for.

If I stay with that reflection and really spend the time to immerse myself in gratitude and begin thinking of the miracles in my life, this practice never fails to turn a negative-trending frequency back up— the right direction! After all, we can't think about two things at once. So we do have the power to change out a negative for a positive.

Our tendency is toward self-criticism and negativity, so positive-trending thought patterns must be consciously cultivated.

Deep Breathing

"Breath turns fear to excitement," I once read. And I've discovered that taking deep breaths when I feel anxiety dissipates it. Breathing is central to yoga practice, and the nice thing about breathing is that it can be done anywhere, anytime, even while you're doing something else.

One of your challenges is to take thirty deep breaths a day. This doesn't just clean out your respiratory system, it also immediately increases your frequencies, and you'll find your mood and energy lifting! When you get to the top of each breath, take one last sip. When you get to the bottom of your exhale, push one more time, eliminating stale carbon dioxide to give yourself a true deep-clean.

On your Resources page, I've made you three different 10-Minute, Five-in-One flows, any of which you can start your day with, to raise your vibe in five different ways at once. One is centered on yoga and a gratitude meditation; the second is a t'ai chi flow; and the third is for clearing negative emotions. Do any of them in the sunshine, while taking 30 deep breaths, and with your feet in the grass, dirt, or sand—and you've done something amazingly beneficial for your ViQ in five different ways!

The Company You Keep: Your Vibe Attracts Your Tribe

You may have heard the saying "Your vibe attracts your tribe," which suggests how powerful the people you allow into your energy field are in raising or lowering your personal frequencies. It's a great learning experience to become mindful of how various people affect you.

People with intuitive abilities who are highly attuned to energetics will often identify and describe very quickly sensing a dark energy, or a light, or a pure force field when in the energy field of another person.

> "Your vibe attracts your tribe."
>
> Unknown

Some refer to auras (somewhat similar in concept to the scientific principle of the vibration of the entire organism), which can range in depth from approximately an arm's length to filling a whole room.

The great energy healer Donna Eden, who says she "sees energies," made this wonderful comment about how she interacts with others' energy fields in her seminal book, *Energy Medicine*:

> When a client's energies are humming, an exquisite, pulsating, captivating scene is laid out in front of me, as if ribbons of energy are moving up and down the body, weaving intricate patterns. The energy pathways are open and spacious rather than dense and congested. Like an endless waterfall, other energies spill up and over the top of the head, and a field of energy surrounds and caresses the body.

Donna Eden has trained many to tap into their inner "intuitive" and begin to see energies we may have been blind to. With all the colorful imagery that those who "see" energies describe, it's no wonder that some auras or energies work with yours and some don't—although that can change, as you make different choices or another person does.

Notice that when someone is in a funk and talking about negatives in their day, they bring your own spirit low.

Have you found that there are people you meet whom you feel you've known forever, and you can't get enough of each other? Others, hopefully much less often, you're literally repelled by, and you may even find yourself rocking back on your heels as they speak.

What kind of frequency are *you* resonating at? If your vibration is low, you will attract others with similar frequencies into your life—your professional life, your social life, and your intimate life. Can you afford this?

If I told you that everyone is attracted to high-vibration people, it wouldn't be true. If you're chronically resonating low, you will find high-energy, creative, positive, happy people downright annoying. You have been aware of this your whole life, whether you've put words to it or not. Your feelings toward them might be described as sarcastic, jealous, or just vaguely frustrated.

I am not suggesting we abandon all suffering and live on the Good Ship *Lollipop*. Pollyanna is in a movie, not real life. And sometimes we must endure hardship and misery and be content and patient with pain and suffering.

However, when a dark spirit troubles you and your intuition tells you an energy coming from a person is not safe, it's important that you be protective of your delicate and sacred holistic vibration. We don't always know why a vibration is harmful to us, but it's important to heed our intuition. After all, you are in the process of cultivating a beautiful harmonic energy. Don't let anyone take it from you.

One of the wonderful things about consciously cleansing yourself energetically of many physical and emotional impurities, is that your social and professional life will improve toward having far more wins and fewer losses.

You invite high vibrations into your relationships and weed out those who don't resonate with you by asking them questions about what's new and wonderful with their lives. I often ask a friend I haven't seen in a while, "What's the best thing in your life right now?"

Everyone loves this question. Sometimes my friend will say, "A bunch of things!" And then I get to explore them, one by one. After I get the lowdown on one great project she's working on or a new relationship she's found, I'll say, "And what else?"

Watch the energy of the person you're with increase as you express genuine enthusiasm for what's going on in her life. And don't stop with just one question. When she answers the first one, if she seems eager to talk, ask a follow-up question: "And what was that like for you?"

A new doctor once expressed his fascination with my medical chart and said, with astonishment in his voice, "What's it like to be you?"

What a wonderful question that is! Everyone has a story and wants to share it. When you invite someone to share their story, you learn so much of great value. Truth is stranger than fiction, and hearing people's real stories can be better than the best of the Harry Potter or Twilight series. Having the discipline to sit with someone's story, encouraging it to unfold, and not rushing it or co-opting it to make it about you—"That happened to me once!"—enriches your relationships by showing deep caring about what matters to someone who enters your energy field.

I remember being so smitten by that question, when my new doctor asked me. And now I love to ask that question, or something like it: What's it like to be you?

Truly listening and showing interest is transformative, because it elevates and lifts everyone you're with. As they listen, others will be wondering, "When will she show such interest in me?" consequently raising the vibe of everyone near you. To have someone listening, fascinated, to your story, your life, is like the sun shining on you. And you have an opportunity to be as resonant and radiant as a ray of sunshine.

Being around positive, self-actualizing people and relationships is one of the most powerful ways to maximize your ViQ.

Who in your life raises your vibe? Most likely it is because that person sees the best in you, sees the best in life, and talks about exciting, interesting things.

Be the change you want to see in the world. If you want to be around more positive people, be more positive. It's that simple. You will attract it as you become it.

Any healthy and happy person over the age of forty will tell you that he has learned that relationships are his most valuable asset and give him the most joy in life. This is true in a career—in almost any profession, we are all deeply connected. But it's also energetically true that we are lifted by each other's frequencies in the form of optimism, encouragement, and authentic love.

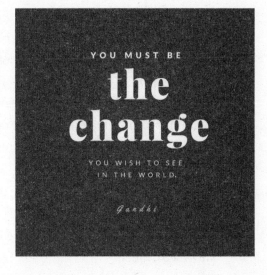

YOU MUST BE

the change

YOU WISH TO SEE IN THE WORLD.

Gandhi

Many of us feel chaotic energies on a crowded New York City street corner and find them mildly distressing. But one-on-one, or in a healthy family where the expression of love is common, we drink deeply from the energies there, and in these relationships we find the strength to go forward with our many challenges. Compassion, love, support, kindness—these matter to the people you encounter far more than the stuff in your brain—facts, data, opinions—that you share with them.

Virtually all high-vibration people have wonderful friendships and have enjoyed a warm and rich tapestry of relationships with partners, colleagues, subordinates, and children—relationships in both life and business. I've noticed that the truly successful may or may not be especially high in IQ—Malcolm Gladwell documents in his book *Outliers* that an IQ of 130 is high enough for someone to accomplish absolutely anything—but those with more emotional intelligence, or EQ (a term coined by Daniel Goleman), and optimized ViQ (my own term) don't just write the most books and develop the most technologies. They also tend to have the most friends and the closest, mutually rewarding relationships.

A high Vibrational Quotient leads you to *all good things*.

In the How High Is Your Vibe? quiz, you were asked about the level of conflict in your relationships. This is not to make a judgment about whether you have disagreements with a spouse or a coworker. The critical point is, does conflict define the relationships—and when conflicts occur, do you resort to silence or violence? Or do you have the difficult conversations and come to a place of more trust, more love, and more respect for each other?

Pets

I wrote most of this book with one of my two cats curled up in my lap or at my feet.

Many research studies show that having a pet (of any kind, whether it's one that sleeps on the bed, in a cage or aquarium, or even in the barn) can positively affect the physical and mental health of adults and children in many ways. It can:

- Lower blood pressure
- Regulate heart rate
- Lower cholesterol
- Increase serotonin
- Relieve depression
- Lower stress and anxiety
- Boost confidence, self-esteem, and empathy
- Relieve chronic pain by releasing endorphins
- Prevent allergies in babies and children
- Decrease behavioral distress in children
- Improve relationships and bring families and friends closer
- Help children without siblings develop emotionally and socially
- Help those who live alone feel less lonely and be more social
- Enhance the elderly's physical well-being and performance of daily living activities.

Mindfulness

In order to become very mindful, I took a twelve-hour course called *Practicing Mindfulness* created by the Rhodes College professor Mark Muesse, which can be purchased on Audible.

The mere act of peeling a tangerine is something he trains you in, to help you become conscious at a very detailed level of everything going on in your world. I love this practice for the way it makes you more finely attuned to the reactions and feelings of others around you, for instance, so you can respond to the needs of your children, your coworkers, your employees, or anyone you care about.

We often operate on autopilot and become oblivious and desensitized to most of the stimuli in our environment. We miss so much of the "juice" in life when we're constantly buzzing and out of tune.

When my friend Alan died suddenly after a week of chemo, his wife, Laura, only forty-eight years old, was given some amazing advice by another young widow who had gone through the process a few years before. She said something you might never expect:

"At the funeral, go to embrace it. Feel every single thing. Drink it in. Absorb all the love you will feel there. Know that this is an event where you will learn so much and feel so much, and lots of it is good and transcends grief. You will always want to keep the memories of this event with you."

I listened to that *Mindfulness* audiobook from the Great Courses while I ran, which is a good multipurposing of my time, and helped me get clear on all the things that matter in my subtle-energetics field. The more mindful I become, the more I feel I can make micro-adjustments with my words, actions, and thoughts to live a consistently higher-vibration life.

"Slow down to speed up." You've heard that saying. It's not accurate to think that to raise vibration we have to speed up! In fact, slowing down—taking even a few minutes for yoga, for meditation, and for tuning in to your inner world—can be profound in grounding you and making you better at everything you do, including functioning in caring relationships. While this may seem counterintuitive, being very still and thoughtful can, in fact, raise your vibe. Grounded frequencies are strong and consistent—and remember, that's every bit as important for optimized ViQ. You aren't living at one frequency, just as you don't have one note to your voice.

Michael Tyrrell's *Wholetones*, which I praise in multiple places in this book (see your Resources page for a link where you can hear samples), is a set of seven twenty-two-minute musical pieces, each constructed around a different healing but perfect frequency. Each has its place. You are more blended, have more character, and are more dimensional than a single note. Optimal ViQ means you live at the beautiful frequencies.

Tapping (or Emotional Freedom Technique)

"Tapping" is a wonderful technique that puts discoveries about the body's energy systems—which are actually ancient discoveries of energy meridians used by Chinese practitioners for two thousand years—very literally under your own fingertips.

Until practitioners began teaching the Emotional Freedom Technique (EFT) about twenty years ago, releasing stuck energies or blockages in the body's energy pathways required the help of acupuncturists and acupressure energy workers. I love that with this technique we can resolve our own blockages, quickly and without any special equipment, with some basic knowledge and practice.

And in seconds, you can turn your energies in a different direction by engaging your mind and moving it to surrender to positives and to releasing.

EFT can be helpful for physical pain and also for emotional pain caused by loss, betrayal, feeling undervalued, stress, and anxiety, as well as the many other ways that you might describe discomfort—all of which, remember, are nothing more nor less than energies.

In addition to tapping on acupressure points in a series, you voice positive affirmations so that both physically and verbally you are moving through, and out of, a negative or stalled space.

A branch of psychotherapy that has become very popular even in traditional therapists' offices is EMDR (short for Eye Movement Desensitization and Reprocessing), which also uses the body's energetic systems to retrain the brain to help clients resolve trauma. Hundreds of published studies show the efficacy of this therapy, which uses kinesthetic sense and eye movement work to change brain frequencies associated with trauma.

One takeaway from EMDR has made its way into what many EFT practitioners teach: if you're tapping on corresponding points on either side of the body, you are advised not to tap both sides in sync, but rather in any erratic pattern that does not match up left to right. This may increase the effectiveness of the technique.

Most traditional EFT practitioners teach you to tap with two fingers, your index and middle fingers. You can use the right or left hand. Since there are usually corresponding tapping points on either side of your body, you can use both hands to tap alternate sides—but if you're using just one hand, it's fine to switch back and forth.

The tapping points start on the top of your head, moving downward on the body, and you should tap on each point approximately half a dozen times, or for about the time it takes you to take one deep breath and release it.

Remove your rings, bracelets, watch, and necklaces, if that's easy in your circumstances, and, if possible, drink a glass of water first, since that facilitates conductivity of electricity. Let's get started trying a tapping pattern, with verbalization, to resolve a negative emotion.

While tapping the following points (with both fingers of both hands), say the sentence on the next page that represents a desire for you related to a low-vibe emotion such as those mentioned above.

TH: Top of head

IEB: Inside Eyebrow

OE: Outside the Eye

UN: Under the Nose

CH: Chin

CB: Collarbone

UA: Under the Arm

WR: Wrist

Sample affirmation: "Even though I have this _____, I deeply and completely love and accept myself."

You don't have to actually believe what you're saying (though that would be nice) for this technique to be efficacious. Now that you're at this point in the book, however, you may find more "belief" in this system of clearing bad vibes that could have seemed bizarre previously.

I remember when my mother bought me an EFT manual when I was in my twenties—I thought it was voodoo and refused to try it. How ironic that I felt it was unscientific and silly, yet what brought me around to it many years later was discovering quantifiable science supporting this and many other practices that shift energies with the mind, or even with manual, physical stimulation—and in this case, both!

If you're in a social setting and can't leave to use this EFT technique when you need a shift in frequencies, do it with one hand and say the words in your mind. People may think you're just trying to remember something!

Many people get relief from physical pain such as headaches using EFT, which shouldn't surprise you, since by now you know that, as Einstein said, "Everything in life is vibration." Including pain.

I've made a video for you on how tapping can help you turn around a fractured vibe and smooth it out. You can find it, with your other resources, on your Resource page.

Mastery of Emotions

It has been a long, difficult, and gratifying journey to move from my childhood of chaos, anger, and fear, to a place of love, acceptance, grace, and peace.

The more I learn about and practice the process I teach in this book, the ninety-second exercise to Metabolize/Reframe/Release any negative emotion (see chapter 2), the happier and more peaceful I become.

This process helps me feel that I am in control of my life, including my feelings, while honoring that feelings are instructive. I think of this process like the old video game Pac-Man.

These ninety seconds you spend can gobble up anxiety, anger, and frustration and put points on your scoreboard! And guess what—you're going to lose that ninety seconds anyway, because when someone flips you off in traffic or undermines your work in a meeting or kicks your child off a sports team, you're going to lose at least ninety seconds of happiness and productivity to those awful feelings, whether you do this process or not!

Mastering your emotions (through the Metabolize/Reframe/Release method) doesn't mean you never feel the negative ones. It means you recognize the learning opportunity, you shift it early rather than late, and negatives become positives, meaningfully and in record time.

I do not "Pollyanna" my feelings, ignoring, stuffing, or faking; however, I also do not allow my high frequency to be hijacked by a negative event for long, or even at all, most of the time.

What am I really feeling, since often the truly legitimate emotion is below the surface of the obvious emotion? What is there to learn from this? How can I do something in this crucible I'm in that is the "opposite" of instinct? How can I live in my higher human functions and honor the divine in not only the other person but myself?

What can I do with this situation for my own growth?

When I ask these questions before choosing to react to a stressful or conflict-oriented situation, large or small, everything that happens to me is opportunity.

This has been a very rewarding journey, to learn this method of keeping my vibration high, regardless of circumstance. I discovered this method through the most difficult three-year period of my life, when many people were depending on me and some of the hardest experiences of my fifty years happened, one after the other, in a series of events that still, when I look back, takes my breath away.

I could not afford to go down. I was a single mother of four children at vulnerable ages who needed me, as well as a business owner with twenty employees who depended on me for income, and many other colleagues associated with me would also be affected by my strength or weakness.

I'm proud to say I'm still standing—stronger and far more compassionate and deep-rooted than before.

My quick metabolism of a negative emotion might sound a bit like an autistic person's reaction, not being aware of others' emotions, if you didn't understand that I am truly experiencing and honoring my own feelings and others', while making meaning of it toward resolution, and doing so quickly.

This is very different from behaving like an automaton and not actually "feeling" much of anything. What I want to teach you isn't that "anything you say bounces off me and sticks on you," a rudimentary way that children on a playground have of responding to a bully. (Which is entirely creative, if you ask me, and appropriate at their level of development for keeping themselves safe in a threatening situation!)

When you Metabolize/Reframe/Release, consider it a full-circle healing of the entire psyche. Consider it your ticket to freedom from bad vibes.

Feng Shui

We have explored so many ways that science has discovered, or is starting to glimpse, the power of energetics. *Feng shui* (pronounced "fung shway") is an ancient Chinese concept, now studied by many all over the world, of harmonizing the physical environment to be conducive to the invisible forces or energies that the Chinese call *qi* (pronounced "chee").

A practitioner of feng shui is educated in sensing *yin* (female, dark) and *yang* (male, light) energies and arranging the environment for balance. Yin and yang refer to opposites, though not gender as we know it. Feng shui practitioners also look for harmony and balance in the five elements of metal, earth, fire, water, and wood.

While some consider feng shui superstitious or outdated, it gives rise to the very solid notion that the arrangement of furniture and art in your home, or the mix of fire, water, metal, wood, and air in your environment, gives it balance and grounding—literally and figuratively—just as these elements are all represented and balanced in nature. Readers also may enjoy and find useful a bit more learning about this Chinese art, for finding balance in their own male and female energies (we all have both, and some of us could develop more of one or the other). Balancing and optimizing energetics may be as important as consistently and gradually increasing energies.

The most fundamental part of creating a positive space is to have your office and home be clean and uncluttered. But if you're looking for more, here are some practical, detailed tips for achieving feng shui in living spaces:

- When looking for a place to live, seek out a home or apartment with views of nature or an uplifting city skyline. Avoid obscured views and views of places like prisons, cemeteries, and industrial areas.
- If you have a choice of floor plan (designing or choosing), it should ideally have good flow to it and make

sense to you. Avoid oddly shaped homes or apartments that make furniture placement and general flow difficult.

• Light and, therefore, windows are extremely important. Natural sunlight is best, but indoor lighting that mimics daylight also helps. But any type of light is better than too little.

• Choose wall paint colors carefully. Bright, vivid colors are best in kitchens. Subdued colors like greens, purples, and blues are best for restful/calming bedrooms. Any color that reminds you of water is a great shade for bathrooms. A shade of white is fine if you don't have the time or "designer skills" to choose colors and combinations for all your walls.

• In general, furniture size in any room should be conducive to the space in the room; avoid overcrowding. Remember to allow for flow, especially in high-traffic areas. The best guideline for general calming is cleanliness and no clutter.

• **Living room:** To promote balance and warmth for groups of people, provide a tight, circular layout (or other communal shape) for chairs and sofas to facilitate conversation. Have a central element to gather around, such as a coffee table, fireplace, or ottoman. Hide televisions, which aren't aesthetically pleasing and can suck the energy out of the room. Place some fresh green plants to help bring in the outdoors. If you have a high ceiling, hang beautiful artwork at eye level to create a focal point and prevent the energy from rising to the ceiling.

• **Bedroom:** To promote relaxation and sensuality, use soft fabrics with a luxurious feel to help the room feel like an escape. Don't place the bed on the same wall as the door, which brings a feeling of insecurity to sleepers. Two bedside tables create a sense of balance. The color palette should be soothing, but hints of pink or red will add a romantic feeling. Any wall art should be calming and positive. Choose mood lighting with dimming features to let you control the feel of the room. Avoid electronics (TV, computer, portable devices) in the room so they don't become the focus of your energies rather than the bed; one exception is a device that provides relaxing and romantic music, which can be very helpful. Never put a work desk in the bedroom!

- **Bathroom:** This room has often been associated with negative energy, but today there are many suggestions for giving it a more positive vibe. Brighten the room as much as possible; if there are no windows, use plenty of great lighting. Add the fire element of candles to offset the overwhelming water elements in the room. If it's a smaller bathroom, use large mirrors to create a sense of openness. Use matching towels for balance and cohesiveness. Keep the drains closed and the toilet lid down to prevent energy from leaving the room. And cleanliness is especially important here, since the bathroom is considered a dirty place.

- **Office/work space:** Although this is the source of your vitality and wealth, it can also be strongly associated with stress. That's why it should always be kept separate from every other room where you live, rest, and play. To increase your productivity, make the desk the focal point. Symmetry throughout the room adds a sense of order and harmony. Live plants purify the air, helping your mind to work better. A small fountain can help calm this normally hectic room. And a clean and uncluttered room helps you work more efficiently.

- **For small/studio apartments:** Try to cordon off the space into "rooms" as best you can, using decorative screens or curtains, especially separating the sleeping and office/work areas. The bed is the piece of furniture that should have the "command position" for the entire apartment space. Keep the entryway open and distinct from the rest of the apartment. If you can paint the walls, use bright, light colors for a more open feeling; strategically placed mirrors will visually expand the space. Keep a balance of furniture and accessories around the entire space, avoiding loud/busy artwork, which will aesthetically crowd the apartment. And use every possible storage space to keep clutter to a minimum.

Sleep

You may think you know what I'm about to say. You're predicting that I'll tell you to get eight hours of sleep every night. In fact, I'm going to tell you something quite different. Eight hours of sleep is just an average.

Just as you shouldn't try to force your child to be the exact average height and weight on the doctor's chart, so, too, sleep is individual. But there are some important principles that will help you be calm, alert, and rested—even if you don't get eight hours of sleep every night.

First of all, an hour of sleep before midnight is worth two hours after midnight! So, even though history shows Ben Franklin didn't walk the talk, he was right about "Early to bed, early to rise, makes a man healthy, wealthy, and wise."

(Caveat: This may not apply to teenagers and young adults, whose circadian rhythms are different from those of older adults and who crave staying up late and waking later in the day. Early morning school is difficult and unnatural for middle and high school students for this reason.)

But going to bed early is a great idea. So is going to bed at approximately the same time every night.

What many people don't know is that the major predictor of whether you're rested isn't how many hours you got. It's whether you were able to complete several sleep cycles. Some people are fine with only four and a half hours of sleep—if they wake up naturally rather than to an alarm clock.

Why does that matter? Because sleep scientists have documented that the natural sleep cycle is about ninety minutes long. When you are unnaturally woken (by an alarm clock or noise) in the middle of a sleep cycle, especially when you are in deeper stages of sleep, you may end up very tired during the day. Then you often end up drinking coffee or other stimulants to get through the day—and you're even more tired the next day. It's a vicious cycle.

Being able to wake up naturally after a ninety-minute sleep cycle is very helpful to your neurological system. And guess how you're more likely to wake up when you're ready to, before your alarm goes off? That's right, by going to bed earlier. And by going to bed at the same time every night.

As you become aware of the ninety-minute sleep cycle and the fact that an hour before midnight is very valuable and restful, take note of whether sometimes you're more rested after six hours of sleep when waking up naturally than after eight hours of sleep when the alarm rouses you.

Natural sleep aids may be of benefit too. They can help you fall asleep quickly, stay asleep, and sleep more deeply and restoratively. I use a dropperful of a fulvic and humic acid supplement (minerals from plant matter decaying in the earth) in water right before bed, and again in a pint of water as soon as I wake up. It keeps my neurological system firing all day, with calm alertness and no need for stimulants.

For a long time, I struggled to get enough sleep and felt anxious every time I didn't get the much-touted eight hours a night. The media had me thinking that if I didn't, I was deficient. When I discovered this amazing concentrated fulvic and humic acid supplement, with all the minerals and trace minerals in perfect balance, I started falling asleep within minutes. Until I discovered this almost ten years ago, it routinely took me an hour or two to fall asleep, so even when I spent eight hours in bed, I got much less sleep than I wanted.

We formulated it because mineral supplements are almost always made from chalks or rocks, and while they're high in minerals, they aren't well absorbed by the body. Fulvic and humic acids come directly from organic sources of ancient plant beds, but before they turn to shale. This is the source that plants used to get their own minerals from, before heavy soil depletion caused by thirty years of pesticide and herbicide use.

Other supplements that have helped many and may be useful to you, depending on what causes your insomnia (there are various reasons), are GABA, valerian root, lavender essential oil, L-theanine amino acid, and, of course, melatonin. (Try not to become dependent on melatonin supplements, or, some experts say, your body will think its job is done and stop producing it naturally at all. Also, try to take just 1 mg or 2 mg doses, not 3 to 5 mg.)

Eight hours of sleep at night may be inferior, then, to seven and a half hours, or even six—if your wake-up involves an interrupted sleep cycle, that is. People who sleep much more than needed have a higher mortality rate—which is to say, you're more likely to die if you sleep too much! (This may not be causal. It may be that grossly overweight people, for example, who are subject to more health issues, sleep more because of lack of energy.)

So there's a range of healthy sleep, and eight hours isn't a magic number. My mother rarely sleeps more than four and a half hours. She'll take a power nap now and then, but her body functions on much less sleep than some others need. You'll get to know your body when you observe these basic principles of getting enough rest.

Achieve Flow States

More than twenty years ago, I read *Flow: The Psychology of Optimal Experience* by psychologist Mihaly Csikszentmihalyi, about research regarding this phenomenal mental state of "flow." In this state, you're so energized, fully involved, and enjoying an activity that you lose track of "self" and you don't notice details in the environment that you're usually aware of.

You've probably experienced it, and when you do, you're in awe of it and wonder how to get back to it more often. In popular vernacular it's called "being in the zone," complete absorption in what you're doing. Another way to think of it is as a "glide pattern."

For me, it often occurs while I'm playing tennis, immersed in a work project such as writing a book, or having a long and extraordinary sexual encounter. You know the feeling: time seems suspended, your every nerve ending seems alive, your creativity is on fire—and afterward you can't believe how much time passed. Because time seemed frozen.

This is actually a great description of what happens when you're in optimal vibration! While this book is about optimizing your electrical energy for fantastic health and happiness, you want to plan for "flow states" as your energetics climb higher and higher—and as they stay high more often and for longer.

So, you're eating cleaner, opting to use positive rather than negative words, and checking your negative thought patterns and replacing them with positives. You're drinking a pint of clean water as soon as you wake up, getting all the electronics away from your bed, and finally going to that yoga class you've been meaning to attend.

Wow, that's six massively powerful habits leading toward a high-vibration life, which is our goal here! So, what will you do with your extra energy, your increased passion, your *joie de vivre*?

Do you remember that great Nikola Tesla quote that I shared with you in the introduction? "If you want to find the secrets of the universe, think in terms of energy, frequency, and vibration."

Do you want to find the secrets of the universe?

What a spectacular question. Tesla wanted to know—more than he wanted happiness, money, or an intimate relationship—the secrets of the universe.

If you responded to that question with indifference, then we're still working with you on the upgrade that is the goal of this book. That's okay. But remember that when you were five years old, you were constantly curious, constantly exploring, with boundless energy and enthusiasm.

What if it's possible to really, truly want the secrets of the universe—once you recover your *joie de vivre*?

This has everything—and I mean everything—to do with raising your ViQ.

Think of the things you used to love to do but don't do anymore. This, my friend, is the great gift of the high-vibration life. Being happier. Doing more of what you love. Spending more time with people you adore—planning a dinner party, setting up a hiking trip, saving some money to go see a few Broadway plays.

Think of all you could do. Get the band back together. Start drawing or painting again. Sign up for a cooking class. Sit down to outline that book you've always wanted to write.

When we are in flow—and I recommend reading *Flow* if you love projects and want to study this concept—we are operating at peak capacity. Every function of our minds and bodies can be fully leveraged. How exciting is that? It's when we are *fully alive*.

Dream, flow, vibrate. It's all in your power—and it's part of your destiny to achieve what you uniquely came to this planet to do.

Live in Today, Plan for the Future

"Live in the moment." "Be present." You've heard these concepts many times, and they're important. I don't think people in the agrarian economy two hundred years ago had to be told to "be present." It's the challenge of living in the twenty-first century, when we are bombarded with social media, electronic productivity tools, devices providing advertising and entertainment . . . messaging and media everywhere.

And many of us, especially white-collar professionals, spend most of our day in front of a computer, where words and images pop out at us constantly. It's a new discipline we've had to develop, to stay on task and be productive, with so many reasons to look at the past (there's an electronic record of it, everywhere!), worry about the future, and slide sideways into time and focus drains.

I'm a big fan of working on your consciousness and being fully present in a project or a conversation. Without that discipline, there is no flow state. Have dinner in a restaurant with friends without checking your cell phone. Talk to your child and look at him throughout the conversation, remembering the social cues that no one had to be reminded of fifty years ago: eye contact, smile, touch.

However, whenever I hear the advice to "stay present, stay in the now," I also think about how many of our modern problems are caused by too little thought for the future—an obsession with the "now."

Some of us need to be called back into the present, particularly those who struggle with depression or anxiety. It is said that depression is an irrational obsession with the past, and anxiety is an obsession with the future. If either of those descriptions resonates with you, then these might be useful practices: bringing yourself fully into the present moment, feeling your feet on the ground, feeling yourself breathe in and out, feeling your eyes moving in their sockets. Anytime you feel that you're coming apart at the seams, yoga, mindfulness, meditation, grounding essential oils, and grounding music all can help you achieve a more centered position.

Learning to be more present may also be helpful if, for instance, you are abrupt with people you care about because it's a pattern for you to be obsessed with time, which seems too scarce, and you're often breathless, rushed, and late to your meetings and social commitments.

But for some, that's not quite the right advice, to "be in the now." Some people suffer needlessly throughout their years by refusing to acknowledge that the consequences of their actions right now will affect their future. If you've started a business but you keep spending your revenues as soon as they come in on travel and play, the time and money drain will eventually cause you to fail. Which will affect your family and your employees, your future opportunities, and even whether you can keep your home.

If you "live in the now" when it comes to food, today's lunch of a quarter-pounder, biggie fries, and a seventy-two-ounce soft drink will take you places today—and in coming weeks, months, and years—that affect everything from your weight to your ability to do your work, from your use of personal time (for sick days instead of fun vacations) to the length and quality of your life.

If you "live in the now" with regard to how you communicate with your partner, in business or in life, you may say things that have an enormous effect on your future with that person. Remember that the vibrations of your heart will register an impact on the heart or brain waves of people physically close to you (and possibly even those emotionally but not physically close at the time). How much more impact, then, does the spoken word have?

How we treat others with our words should be given thought with regard to the future of that relationship. Speaking clearly and speaking compassionately are not mutually exclusive. Remember that the great communicators of the business world and the personal growth field do both simultaneously.

So each approach is appropriate at different times: tuning in and grounding yourself in the now, as well as delaying gratification for our own and others' future interests. The high-vibration human learns to recognize when to rein in anxiety and scattered vibes with a grounding exercise. He also knows when to put off pleasure or sleep or travel to focus instead on work that makes next month or next year a bright place for him, his family, and the world around him.

Tapping into Your Unconscious: Dream Work

My good friend Machiel Klerk is a renowned psychoanalyst and Jungian dream analyst. I first met him when I attended his lecture and discovered the concept of dream work. That is, rather than just dreaming and looking up meanings in an online dream symbols dictionary, which may or may not have any relevance to you, you can actually use your dreams to understand and resolve issues blocking energy in your conscious life.

Which means instead of shrugging your shoulders about how weird and inexplicable your dreams are, ask your dreams for help! Machiel tells his clients to keep a dream journal, a notebook beside the bed. Much like the ritual of praying at night right before bed, your ritual in keeping a dream journal is to write down questions you want to solve or learn about, and then go to sleep with those things on your mind.

The conscious and unconscious are very much linked. We know this because many of us have had dreams featuring snakes, falling, flying, or having sex with a person we have no conscious attraction to. Even if you believe that the theories of Freud and his student Jung have validity, they are not the final authorities on what *your* dreams mean for *you*.

Our dreams can contain clues regarding where our energies may be stuck in our progress toward higher symphonic vibrations. Instead of thinking of your dreams as a bizarre mystery, consider them to be a possible doorway to things your subconscious is trying to tell you.

Letting Go of What Doesn't Serve

Many years ago, when I was pushing hard to make a trip to a trade show in New York City happen that just wasn't coming together (everything going wrong despite a huge amount of effort), I was asked by a wise person:

"Robyn, do you ever wonder, when things are too hard, if it isn't meant to be?"

As someone who prides myself on being able to do hard things, that was a pattern interrupt I needed. The permission to quit.

It simply is not how my brain works, to give up, and my natural tendency is to dig in harder as circumstances conspire against me. But sometimes giving up is the perfect thing to do, and we just need permission to let go. We hear "never, ever give up" so often, but sometimes the perfect thing to do is just that: to quit. To stop doing things that aren't "great." To put our energy elsewhere.

Not to give up on our children. Not on our health. Not on our most cherished dreams. Not on self-love.

But it's okay to let go of something that didn't work. It's even okay to change your dreams.

Quitting allows you to switch directions, opening a door to change and grow and redeem something of value. Quitting lets you reinvent—including reinventing yourself!

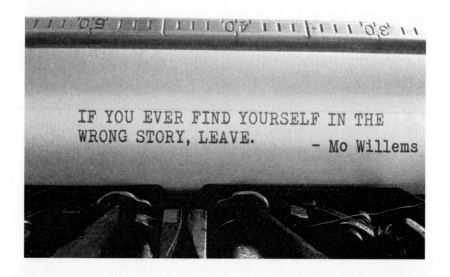

IF YOU EVER FIND YOURSELF IN THE WRONG STORY, LEAVE. — Mo Willems

Eight years past my divorce, if I'm in a conversation with a newly divorced person, I often volunteer to serve as a "divorce spirit guide," since it is a long and difficult transition, especially for someone who, like me, was married for more than twenty years—my entire adult life, at the time of that major change.

And the first and most important lesson I've learned that I share with a divorce newbie is to let go. Let go faster, and with grace, of negative emotions, of attaching to outcomes, of feeling that your children's every opinion and every decision is a reflection on you. Let go of dwelling on your mistakes.

Let go of the need to be perfect. Let go of feeling like what happened today matters so much in the long run. Let go of what others think of you.

My own "spirit guide," Matthew Flinders, was a couple years ahead of me in his divorce process. He said, "When you find yourself getting overwrought about something, ask yourself: Will this matter in a year?"

I've found that the answer to this is almost always no! And that reminds me of the book Matthew had me read back then, Richard Carlson's *Don't Sweat the Small Stuff . . . and It's All Small Stuff*.

Ironically, and sadly, Richard Carlson died suddenly not long after his books were published, in his forties, leaving two young daughters behind. I interviewed his wife on my podcast, *Your High-Vibration Life*, about how little the minutiae of life matter when you die. Carlson's life and death exemplify what he taught.

It makes all the difference in your ViQ to let go faster than slower—clinging to a plan, a belief, a failed venture, or a relationship—as soon as you realize it does not serve you or others.

Sexual Energetics—the Most Powerful Force Field in the Universe

How you use your sexuality has everything to do with your overall Vibrational Quotient. It would be easy to leave that subject out of this book, as it is not discussed very often in polite or academic conversations.

But it needs to be addressed. It's no secret that many otherwise smart, high-functioning people have sex and intimacy confused. The market for therapy and treatment for "sex addicts" is rising, as more light is shined on this phenomenon and pornography of every type imaginable is available at the touch of anyone's fingertips. The addicts themselves suffer at least as much as their partners do, with the loss of more authentic connection and, often, actual physical sexual dysfunction.

You could argue that the power to give life to another human being, or to participate in that act regardless of whether it culminates there, is the most significant power that regular human beings ever witness and are part of. In fact, orgasm and conception are virtually simultaneous!

But what is the act that initiates the orgasm? The act of sexual intercourse is likely the most intense form of energy exchange there is. Women describe being literally "pounded," and we should acknowledge here the damage that can occur to an energetically sensitive person—and, in fact, any of us, as we are all sensitive—when we don't understand and honor the power of that exchange.

This suggests how careful we must be, in a world where "sexual liberation" is taken for granted and sex is trivialized, to allow this mingling of energies only when we know and trust our partner, we feel safe, and we are resonating on a similar wavelength.

Sometimes one partner in a dance-for-two uses sex to try to level disparate frequencies when there has been an energetic disconnect. This is generally ineffective as relationship repair and can, in fact, deepen the divide, since sex is simply the manifestation of the connection—not the other way around.

It can take an extended period of time for a sensitive person to recover from a low-vibration sexual interaction. We know this intuitively, as it is an act the vast majority of us engage in only highly selectively, regardless of religious background. The average person has an average of only four partners in a lifetime.

Archetypally, women have had, throughout history, one of two roles: one as a prostitute, sexual object, or sexual privilege (for profit and pleasure); and, two, as a mother (or breeder). In order to achieve anything beyond those two roles, a woman has, historically, needed to adopt "male" traits, to behave like a man.

This has been the modern woman's uphill battle, to break into other "power" roles. When I was twenty years old and got married in conservative Utah, I chose to hyphenate my name; my own family (and his) told me, disdainfully, "Keeping your name is not your right, it's your brothers'!" and "You're clearly not ready for the commitment of marriage."

Very recent history (the past two generations) has altered the popularity of the sexual archetypes, although they are still very familiar to all of us and are alive and well, while somewhat underground. Those of us living the modern fantasy of empowerment for women are the beneficiaries of updated social norms and opportunities, but we also have all the confusion of those vibes around our historical past, regarding roles and sexuality, to work through.

Generally speaking, those archetypes are that the male is the pursuer and the female is the pursued: the resistant partner, the submissive—even the sedated! (Men have sedated women for sexual purposes since the dawn of time.)

My own grandfather, when he performed marriage ceremonies, used to refer to "wifely duties," a concept that divides older from younger generations. Since the women's movement and the sexual revolution, it is no longer in vogue for women to admit to, or relish, or even talk about roles such as "the submissive" in sexuality or in any other arena.

Some of the world's religions forbid sexuality, and virtually all of them attempt to police it and restrain it. Some individuals (including our dear Nikola Tesla, around whose discoveries this book revolves) choose to metaphorically castrate themselves—although I refer specifically to monks, priests, and nuns, who deny their own sexuality because it is base or carnal, and they feel called to spirituality and divinity, long considered to be higher realms of consciousness. Our collective past is rich with examples of the idea that higher states of being and the sex act are mutually exclusive.

I believe that part of the reason we have so many conflicted feelings about our own sexuality stems from the male perspective that orgasm is the whole point in the bedroom.

Orgasm is the point of conception, and we spend the rest of our lives seeking it again, and so sexuality is a highly manipulated experience where the male (archetypally) seeks to make the experience whatever results in an orgasm for him.

The most a woman can hope for—and fortunately it is common in the modern age—is that he wants her to have the same experience: he cares that she has the "destination experience," the orgasm. Men have been taught that they should care about their partners' orgasms, and many of them pride themselves on helping their partner achieve it through various means.

They believe that orgasm is the holy grail of sex.

But what if it is just a stepping-stone toward a far more evolved state of sexual intimacy? What if the "revolution" of the female orgasm, the fact that it's socially acceptable for women to seek pleasure in the experience as well, is just one point along the path?

A few men are realizing that sex can be a journey rather than an event to be manipulated for orgasm as the concentration of all points of light (frequencies) for the ultimate destination. When they discover this, they tap into a set of frequencies that are grounded and giving (rather than receiving). A man fully committed to this potentially experiences a transcendent sexual and overall relationship, because he has accomplished the ultimate in female submission:

He thinks that "ultimate" is to orgasm. He's wrong. The ultimate for her, his job in the bedroom, is to make her feel both safe and loved.

Orgasm is the highest frequency we can bring into the physical dimension. But when we allow ourselves to tap the resonance of a "journey" sexual experience instead of the "destination" of the orgasm-driven experience, which we'll talk about in this section, it can transport us to a different level of intimacy.

Sometimes when we experience tremendously powerful frequencies during a period of elation, a period of depression can follow. This high-vibing experience (and subsequent crash) can come via any of the experiences we discuss in this book, but it's never more likely than with a powerful sexual experience.

That's because that ecstatic experience brings up your emotional blockages, unearthed by the electricity of your sexual experience. (Remember, a high rate of oscillation can detoxify a cell—so it stands to reason that same high vibe is going to dislodge some discomfort and some pain points in a relationship. In effect, it can detoxify you—if you allow for the emotional reaction and sit with the pain points it brings up and embrace the process.)

After all, any good "energy healer" will tell you after your session to expect some emotional fallout, volatility, colorful dreaming, and other subconscious reactions to a major shift in your energies.

So sex can be therapeutic not just because it feels good and causes a release (orgasm and oxytocin are good for you!), and because it can be deeply intimate and loving, but also because it can identify some of the lower frequencies you may want to bring into the light and address.

Thus, after a profound sexual experience, couples often report conflicts over small things in the ensuing days. In some relationships, it can even result in a breakup or one partner pulling back—and she doesn't even know why.

If this has happened to you, and it's mystifying and frustrating, just know that this is energetics playing out, and they can be resolved. If we become reflective about the causes, we identify personal and relationship blockages, and this can be a gift in a relationship!

So sex isn't just for making babies, and it isn't just for releasing tension or "getting off." And you probably have a modern enough consciousness to know that it isn't innately "sinful"—I hope so, because throughout time, the religions that ban or vilify sex just drive it underground and cause it to take sinister forms.

In fact, certain types of sexual experiences can be a profoundly powerful healing tool, because merged vibrations are so heightened and so very intimate.

"Orgasmobiles" is how women are often seen by the men who hunt them, Michael Brown says in his book *The Presence Process*. He discusses how energies shift as the male partner removes orgasm as the end goal and decides in advance that he will stop or change anything in the sexual experience when it gets too close to orgasm for him.

He will have a "journey" rather than a "destination" experience, which may positively transform his relationships—not just with his partner, but with all women and all human beings. And Brown recommends putting several days in between sexual encounters, for the low vibes to come out and be worked through between sexual experiences.

The job of the archetypal male aggressor has been to make the world safe for dependents, such as a woman and children.

My twenty-two-year-old daughter, Emma, scrapes her pennies together and heads off for another continent every summer. She works two jobs and lives frugally, saving for her adventures—and every time she leaves, her father and I are terrified.

Because she does not know what an unsafe world it is for her gender. Recently she texted me from Greece, excited to show photos of her on a sailboat with two older men. Because she paid them and because they do this work professionally, she believed herself and her friend to be completely safe out on the water—two female college students with two older, male strangers.

You don't even have to be a parent to have the same reaction I did. Her father and I were losing our minds and calling her, all but shrieking, "Have you seen the movie *Taken*?"

(Or *Taken II*, for that matter? I've seen both, which adds to my anxiety as Emma heads out on one of her adventures. Liam Neeson unleashes superhuman powers to extricate his daughter from a sex-trafficking operation that kidnaps her while she travels with a friend in Europe. I don't sleep well at night when she goes on her couch-surfing foreign trips. "But, Mom!" she says. "There's a couch-surfing *website*, and people we stay with have *ratings!*")

The world isn't particularly safe for women, and the reasons for that run bone-deep, and, in fact, are contained in our DNA. Because women, since getting booted from the Garden of Eden, have frequently found ourselves in vulnerable situations.

A friend of mine read the first draft of this chapter, and what she said in response was indicative. She is married to a committed, good man who loves her. But even for her, the response was, "I'm not sure I want him looking into my soul!"

Many would read my friend's comment and their thought would go to the archetype: men want sex more, and women resist. My mind goes to: "She must not feel entirely safe."

And if, even in committed relationships, we women feel "hunted" and like objects of desire with the never-ending quest for orgasm as the goal, it defines and limits the sexual relationship.

How many marriages do you think have ended in part because a man did not realize that his job in the relationship was to make the woman feel safe and loved (and failed to do so)?

All of this has roots in thousands of years of human sexual behavior, all of your ancestors' consciousness and behavior coming to play in the very *charge* of your DNA. So there's no need to feel guilty about it, if it's a revelation to you that most sexuality is limited and limiting by definition.

However, a transcendent experience completely different from your personal experience thus far is entirely possible! We're going to explore the art of tantra, because I believe it embodies that potential to "use" sex for a different and higher cause: that is, exploring the high sexual vibrations for awareness, healing, and stronger connection.

This is very different than "using" your partner for sex and love to achieve a selfish goal.

Let's back up a bit and talk about the energetics of touch. My friend Dallas Hartwig, coauthor of *The Whole 30*, says of the modern age soaked in electronic communication, "We're all oversexed and undertouched."

Touch is powerfully healing, as much science has shown us, including for newborn infants. Infants who are touched more have much higher positive life outcomes than infants whose basic needs are met but who are not touched often, as is the case in some orphanages as well as in families. It's been shown that especially for newborns, skin-to-skin contact helps to calm them, and they cry less and sleep better. It also facilitates their brain development, and they are at lower risk for emotional, behavioral, and social problems as they grow up.

Transactional sexual experiences with chaotic frequencies are common, and they can be jarring to the whole organism well beyond the event itself. Disturbed and disconnected frequencies collide when one or both partners are under the influence of a substance, when they do not know each other prior to the encounter, when one partner is paid for the transaction or is nonconsenting, or when there is no love or trust in the interaction.

There is a significant amount of touch in most sexual interactions between people who love each other, and there is far less touch in sex between strangers or sex while under the influence of a substance.

Fully half of us are single, even in midlife, an age when people were far more likely to be married a century ago—and social media has replaced much of what used to be our social life.

Porn is ubiquitous and makes up a huge percentage of the commerce on the Internet. A 2008 study showed that 93 percent of boys and 62 percent of girls were significantly exposed to pornography before age eighteen. In 2010, one extensive study discovered that out of the 1 million most popular websites in the world, 4 percent (42,000+) were sex-related, and about 13 percent of web searches were for erotic content. It also found that the five most popular porn sites got 7 to 16 million (individual, nonrepeat) visitors a month, with the most popular site getting 32 million visitors a month—which constitutes almost 2.5 percent of all Internet users.

Regardless of whether you feel pornography has a viable and healthy purpose or you think it has caused the degeneracy of the modern-day Sodom and Gomorrah, which are two ends of the spectrum on how you might view it, there's an epidemic of sexual dysfunction, as some men have now been exposed to thousands of hours of pornography that affect their ability to, if I may be graphic, get an erection, maintain an erection, or complete an orgasm.

Reconnecting sexual practice to the beautiful, powerful, and positive energetic that I believe it was meant to be is the purpose of this section.

As a former practitioner of sex therapy, I loved the ancient practice of tantric sexuality brought into the modern day. You don't have to immerse yourself in Eastern mysticism to find it appealing, if you're looking for a very slow and sensuous experience that doesn't skip over the most delicious part of the sex act.

I feel it's the perfect antidote to an affluent world that craves connection. It's a "journey" rather than a "destination."

I often asked clients: "What's the only thing that's better than sex?"

Mostly they'd look at me, stupefied. The men couldn't think of anything, and the women often ventured, "Chocolate?"

Nope. I'd supply the answer:

"Sexual tension is often even better than sex."

Were it not so, there would be no foreplay and none of the endless jokes among women about their partners' rush to the finish line in the bedroom.

In this porn-saturated world, we have some false and disturbing realities presented to us in literally millions of hours of filmed prostitution available to virtually anyone with a credit card. And much of it is, in fact, available for free, where our children find it.

Filmmakers instruct the actors to keep their hands out of the frame, as the entire scene is shot with the focus on penetration. So foreplay, and anything in sexuality that requires the sense of touch or use of the hands, is mostly taboo.

Pleasure and orgasm are in all the wrong places in pornographic depictions of sex, and an adolescent or adult male would be very confused indeed upon entering his first real sexual experience if he'd received his education from the porn industry.

After all, in porn films a woman administering a blow job often has an orgasm while doing it. (Which makes no sense, biologically.)

Very little of the "story" around a sex act is ever shown. (Unless the pornography was shot for a female audience—in which case, it's low-budget and corny, the narrative that ensues is neither believable nor interesting, and the sex acts substitute for the real-life long, slow play of a woman getting to know a man.)

The fact is, in real life there's always a narrative that leads up to any memorable intimate experience. You imagine the situation before it happens and, in fact, you're likely to dwell on those anticipated details for far longer than the actual event ends up taking.

You plan what you'll wear. You imagine the unfolding of a conversation and a long orchestration of the sexual encounter. Flirting takes place, often for days or weeks, prior to the event itself. The imagination runs wild and makes the event itself even more exciting.

Of course, what actually happens is often very different than what you imagined—after all, two people's narratives and motives may be different. (Which is just one of the reasons I suggest that we be very careful with our sexual energies and recognize the power of them—including the power to be deeply hurt, both men and women.) But that's what's so exciting about it. You are only half the narrative.

To be open to a more meaningful sexual energy, you're going to have to let go of the idea that sex is an emergency.

I mentioned earlier that a friend of mine read this chapter and said, "I'm not sure married people can pull this off—and I'm not sure I want anyone looking at my soul!" She asked if she was an anomaly— and, of course, she's not. I'd pitched my agent on another book I wanted to write, about the connection between diet and good sex, and she didn't want to sell it.

As I talked to other wellness authors, asking their opinion on my book proposal, they told me what I already knew from my previous professional experience. My friend Tami Meraglia, MD, a doctor who works with women in midlife, said: "Women aren't going to buy a book about sex, because their libido is too low and their partners aren't happy about it, but they're just fine with it. It's not bothering *women!*"

If either of those scenarios describes you, we've got some work to do here, in general, with your energetics. (That is, if you relate to my married friend saying she's too exhausted for soul-gazing, or if your partner isn't happy with your libido but you don't much care.)

So I'd love to see you choose from among the ideas in this book to increase your overall energy and ground your frequencies, including doing the 7-Day Detox. This will show up in your sex life, in a positive and powerful way! And that, of course, makes for a very connected and loving relationship.

Late night hours aren't conducive to a good sexual connection for many people. We may have it all wrong, here in the Western world, with this unwritten cultural rule that sex happens at bed-time. This depends on your biorhythms, but think about it: late at night, melatonin production is increasing and the body is preparing for sleep, and suddenly we decide it's a good time to do the most powerfully energetic thing there is, short of running sprints?

The gym is empty at 11 p.m.—because no one wants to run sprints then!

In some cultures of the world, people go home for lunch and make love, because they intuitively realize this. (Those are the same cultures whose people who don't eat a big dinner, and they live longer than we do!)

Sometimes a sexual disconnect in a marriage can be related to different biorhythms, which of course are just a type of vibration. One partner might be a "morning person" who bounces out of bed, ready to go for a four-mile run, and he's married to a person who hits the snooze button three times and needs coffee before a conversation is even possible.

The more detailed *Design Your High-Vibration Life* course that you can learn about on your Resources page has a module on tantric sex, which is beyond the scope of this book. It may read a bit like erotica, but it actually has very little literal sex in it. It's more about structuring and exploring the slow pace of erotic buildup of sexual tension. Few would argue that this isn't the best kind of sex, anyway—but as with everything else in our whirlwind culture, we've lost the art of stillness, the pleasure of grounding, the delicious mystery of exploration.

We all want more connection. When a human being watches porn for the first time, he never realizes that it may harm his ability to create a meaningful and loving sexual relationship.

This process here of tuning in to sexual frequencies is simple, it's as loving as it is erotic, and it's designed to create more electricity in your intimate life and more wellness in your life overall.

Far Eastern Grounding Practices

Yoga

You may have heard this saying common among yogis: "Doing yoga three times a week will change your body. Doing yoga daily will change your life."

Many studies show that yoga is a highly effective practice for connecting your mind to your breath and becoming more grounded, which has everything to do with living a more centered, peaceful, and purposeful life from the frontal lobe of your brain, rather than operating from your emotional, scattered, limbic brain.

Plus, the condition of your spine is key in how quickly you age. Too many of us are sedentary, and many of us sit at a computer all day. I go to yoga class a few times a week, but if I miss it because of work or tennis, I also make a practice of doing yoga poses while I'm in a phone meeting or between games during tennis practice or in airport waiting rooms, rather than sitting in a chair with my spine slowly compressing.

It has changed my health significantly, because I had back and neck pain for decades following a car accident when I was five years old.

In my twenties, I used to wake up sometimes in so much neck pain that I couldn't go to work.

I started doing yoga regularly almost ten years ago, and I have never had neck and back pain again.

On your Resources page, I've shared with you three videos, including a 10-minute yoga flow, to get the most vibration-raising juice out of 10 minutes a day. All you have to do is follow any of the three videos, while taking 30 deep breaths, enjoying the sunshine to charge your battery, and grounding to dump excess negative energies with your feet in the grass or dirt. (Enjoy this daily ritual with someone you love, or a pet, and you've got yourself a sixth, bonus frequency-increasing practice!)

I know it's a big "ask" to suggest you add a ten-minute habit to your day. So I suggest you attach it to another activity. If you exercise, add this ten minutes to the beginning of it. If you have a breakfast ritual or a before-bed ritual, perhaps this belongs there. I'll explain in the next section in detail. But meantime, I want to share with you (if you're not already doing yoga as a regular practice) why it has the power to change not only your health but, even more than that, your peace and happiness.

It's not just the stretching, which makes you limber and more youthful, because your spine slowly becoming calcified is what first ages you. This, to be sure, is an important result of regular yoga—but yoga is half stretching and half stability. We don't think about physical stability much until we lose it. (For many elderly folks, the loss of stability combined with easily broken bones from osteoporosis or osteopenia creates a perfect storm for falls causing serious injury, which is the beginning of the end for many people over eighty.)

Physical stability is dramatically improved for those who do yoga, but there is a powerful mind-body connection that yogis will often tell you about—"stability" is more than just physical. While we don't often think about physical stability in our younger years because we take it for granted, we do see lack of stability all around us as a metaphorical way of describing a sense of our loss of control, volatile emotions, or feeling the ground shifting underneath us.

Yoga has helped ground me in feeling peaceful about "what is," just as much as my physical stability has improved from spending so much time in dancer, downward dog, and triangle poses.

Other benefits of yoga include becoming more centered, becoming more mindful, and developing good breathing habits. A good yoga teacher will help you focus on your breath, synchronizing it to movement (inhale on the way down, exhale on the exertion). This requires you to go deep inside and focus, and you'll find that this mindfulness migrates deeply into the rest of your life.

Plus, yoga teachers are trained in Eastern ways of thinking, and I've heard many aphorisms during yoga practice that really make me think deeply (during yoga is the perfect time for that). These sayings are applicable to living a centered life and have increased my ViQ over the years.

If you dislike yoga the first time you try it, trust the process and give it ten times before you judge. As I went through a divorce after twenty years of marriage, yoga saved me. People say that their friends or their faith or some other saving grace helped them through a divorce—for me, it was yoga and good nutrition! Many people don't like yoga at first and find it uncomfortable. That will change, I promise, if you do it at least three times a week for thirty minutes. The more uncomfortable you find it as you start, the more you need it!

And if you can't devote an entire hour to a yoga class, no worries: you can do short yoga flows you find on YouTube or using various apps. After a few years of practice, you know the poses and balances and flows, and you can listen to what your body wants to do and do it yourself.

Developing balance—for instance, so that you can stand on your right foot with your left hand holding your left foot behind you and your body led by your right arm reaching forward—is extremely helpful as you age. Elderly people often lose their equilibrium and fall. Broken bones, especially hip fractures, can lead to hospitalizations, pneumonia, and other consequences—and yoga is good for your bones, your joints, and your balance.

When you have strong physical balance, interestingly, that leads to its metaphysical corollary as well—a "balanced" mindset in which typical negative events or challenges in the course of your day do not tip you over emotionally.

If you haven't yet discovered the magic of yoga, let me give you one more reason to do so: it will ground and center your vibrations to help you with calm, focus, and an overall feeling of wellness.

Qigong and T'ai Chi

Other Eastern practices such as qigong (or chi-gong) and t'ai chi have effects similar to yoga.

Qigong focuses on breath work while also using meditation and very slow, gentle physical movements to help you imagine energy flowing through your body. This can help calm your nerves, reduce your stress, and lower your heartbeat and respiration rate. It also improves strength and movement.

T'ai chi is similar to qigong in many ways. It offers the same meditation and breathing practice as well as slow, calming movements. This, of course, results in similar benefits to the nervous, cardio, and respiratory systems. It also can improve strength, balance, and flexibility—but whereas qigong is better suited for older people because of its more gentle and less intense movements, t'ai chi's slightly more intense aerobic element makes it a better choice for young and middle-aged participants, as well as older people who are in generally more robust health.

My friend Joe, a t'ai chi master, made a twenty-minute empowerment video for you, to start using these techniques. Don't forget that when you do them, whenever possible, you should go out in the grass barefoot, in the sun, and take deep breaths! The video is on your Resources page.

Meditations

Your ViQ-Raising 10-Minute, Five-in-One Yogic Meditation

In the case of vibration, sometimes you need to slow down to speed up.

I promise, the ten minutes I'm about to describe to you, if practiced daily, can result in far more that you get done.

Adding this to your day is a net gain for you, not a ten-minute loss! It's actually true that sometimes you can spend time to gain time, as with many of the things you learn about here. One way to think of that is by imagining the time you spend doing any of these things as an investment. Money under your mattress loses value; money invested earns interest. The same goes for time.

Think of these habits as an investment in yourself. Time marches on, but if you synergize and "clean" your energies, you'll be far happier and you'll get more done with the time you have available.

And what I'm about to tell you, I'll also show you if you follow the link on your Resources page to a video I've made for you. You can watch and listen as you do it, until you have it memorized.

You're multitasking to do five different upvibing things at the same time—all in just ten minutes. That's obviously a lot of things to do at once—and, in fact, there's a sixth and even a seventh high-vibe practice you can add, when you've got this whole practice down cold. I'll explain that in a minute.

And don't worry if you can't do all five at once in the beginning. You'll get it. Do a few, whichever ones interest you most, and add more as you get comfortable with this. And it's easier than it sounds, because two of them—standing in the grass or dirt getting grounded, and soaking up vitamin D from sunshine on your skin—take no effort at all.

You're going to do yoga with a meditation you can say along with me in the video or while taking thirty deep breaths, getting some sunshine, and grounding your electrical system.

You'll want to do the exercise outside if at all possible, though doing it inside is absolutely better than not at all.

You're going to find a grassy spot, and preferably go outside between 8 a.m. and 10 a.m., but anytime there is sunlight will work, because one of your objectives is sun exposure and soaking up some vitamin D, which keeps your bones strong, prevents cancer, and increases your endorphins.

You're going to be doing some yoga flows while saying a meditation. I like to say the words out loud, because I am less likely to wander off into other thoughts that way. But saying the words in your mind has the same energetic effect.

In developing this meditation, I have been influenced by the great Buddhas and principles taught by the modern Buddhists, as well as by the work of many other teachers who helped me to heal from my traumatic past and to ground and uplevel my own vibe.

Another feature to this exercise is that for as much of it as possible, especially after you practice this a few times, you can close your eyes. This is wonderfully restful, to spend a few minutes each day with your eyes closed. In fact, one study showed that simply closing your eyes for ten minutes a day has restorative and restful benefits akin to taking a nap!

You're also going to take long, slow, deep breaths—thirty of them is perfect—and take your time with them. As soon as one breath feels like you've reached the very top of your lungs, pause for a moment and then sip just a little more air. Do the same at the bottom of an exhale: when you think all the air is gone, stop, and a second later, push out a bit more stale air.

It's in those last bits of breath that you're really vacuuming out the dirty stuff in the respiratory system and bringing in cleansing fresh air and oxygen.

The meditation is designed to assist in your desire to create an improved experience in your life, something more marvelous than you've ever attained before. And after these ten minutes, you should be able to return to work with an altered state, vibrating at least 10 hertz higher!

Over time, meditating literally changes your brain chemistry and makes you more creative, more of a problem solver, more even-keeled emotionally, and more electrically consistent, even under stress. The key is daily practice.

I've written a meditation dedicated to your realizing and achieving your highest and best purpose. You'll want to see the yoga flow we've given you, with music and the meditation playing in the background, and download the one-page PDF of this meditation from your Resources page. You can read from it or refer to it until it's committed to memory, or even just keep the video and play it every day.

Put your device three feet away, with the sound turned up loud enough to hear, so that any negative electromagnetic frequencies do not affect you.

Say the meditation as you do the yoga stretches—and if you're outside with your feet on the ground, "earthing" and discharging electrons into the ground, and recharging your battery in the sunshine, and breathing oxygen taking deep breaths.

And it doesn't matter whether you get the words exactly right. You are simply creating soft and upleveling vibrations with your words and thought frequencies while focusing on healthy thoughts and the powerful emotions of love and gratitude in the meditation.

You're practicing each day to keep focus, which quiets the "chattery monkey" in your brain that fragments your frequency.

Later you can add two bonus practices to the five practices here. First, I invite my pets to my outdoor yoga/meditation/deep-breathing exercises. They're invited because they're helping me transition out of the sympathetic nervous system and into the calming vibes from the parasympathetic system, because I love them, and because they help keep my blood pressure low too!

And I highly recommend that you play one of the *Wholetones* high-vibration CDs or digital recordings that you can download to your device. I've linked you to these seven beautiful pieces, written to 528 Hz and other frequencies by composer Michael Tyrrell, on your Resources page as well, and I encourage you to listen to the samples. We discuss what "high-vibration music" is in just a few more pages. The music is a magical addition to your ten-minute meditative yoga practice.

If your pet or someone you love joins you and you add some high-vibration music, you've actually got seven great things going for you in this short practice!

Infrared Sauna and Physical Detoxing

Worth saving for, a deep-penetrating infrared sauna in a corner of a room, or even a garage or patio, costs less than you might imagine and can be powerful for weight loss, improving circulation and cardiovascular health, and cleansing cells of toxins that have built up.

Cleansing your cells allows them more sensitivity and more ability to increase in oscillation speed.

And, unlike the old-fashioned steam rooms or heat saunas working only on the surface of your skin, infrared has healing frequencies that penetrate deeply, one to two inches, which is detoxifying at an organ level to some extent and is very helpful to the respiratory and cardiovascular systems. In fact, it's a passive cardio workout, as you'll find your heart rate increased at the end of your twenty- or thirty-minute session.

I also do my meditations and breathing exercises there, and take along a book, music, or a podcast to edify me and help justify the time I spend in this "home sanctuary" that is worth every penny I paid for it. If you don't have your own, you can pay for a session in a spa in this helpful device (about $25 an hour) that can give you an accelerated detoxification experience whenever you feel you need it.

The Frequencies of Music

All shape is rooted in vibration, and sound is frequency. So it shouldn't be surprising that there are few things that change your energy faster than music—for good or for bad. Within seconds, you can move from a low-energy state to a higher-energy state simply by choosing a style of music, an artist, or a song that has positive associations for you.

For most people, grounding music is likely more appropriate for doing grounded work that requires thoughtfulness and intellect, unlike the physical energy of a five-mile run. Music types are as varied as people are, but classical, new age, jazz, and many others are soothing to the nervous system and allow most people to get "in the zone" to do their very best work in harmonic vibration. I will go through some examples in this section about how our associations with music affect our vibration, so how we react to certain types of music is highly individual.

Great debate, and a very interesting history, swirls around the frequency to which a stringed instrument is tuned. For many years now, the frequency 440 Hz, or the note A when a string is vibrating at that frequency, has been the tuning standard. If the resonant frequency of the guitar itself is 440 Hz, then when the A string is plucked, the entire guitar will shake.

Remember the Beach Boys song "Good Vibrations," in which Brian Wilson sings, "I'm pickin' up good vibrations . . . she's giving me excitations?" If someone is receiving your good vibrations, it's because you're sending them!

A pure frequency is known as a signal, whereas chaotic or fractured frequencies, in the realm of detectable sound, are called noise. (You may have been trapped in an elevator or on hold on the phone with a musical loop that isn't quite tuned in—isn't it amazing how listening to that "noise" can be almost unbearable and destroys the "clear signal" of the musical notes?)

There are frequencies that are so magical and perfect that Michael Tyrrell (whom I'll tell you more about in a minute) wrote music to the healing frequencies, the frequency of our living planet in all its perfection.

In particular, the 528 Hz frequency of his third piece is more studied and worshipped by artists and scientists than any other frequency. This oscillation is known for its medical laser uses in actually repairing human DNA. It is the frequency of earth, and of living green things, and of the tone *mi* in the seven-note fixed-*do* solfeggio.

There are also frequencies so dissonant, so chaotic to the human brain, that Dr. Leonard Horowitz says that if the 440 Hz frequency were blared from sirens, there would be "mass hysteria in the streets." And Joseph Goebbels—Adolph Hitler's right hand and Nazi propaganda minister who killed himself, his wife, and his six children when Hitler committed suicide—led the effort to internationally institutionalize 440 Hz = A. (He had already made it the official

German pitch, after centuries of 256 Hz = C being the official tuning standard.)

The musical frequency that is the greenish-yellow hue displayed in the plant kingdom, C = 528 Hz, is known to calm emotional distress and possibly even heal human DNA. (If this seems hard to believe, consider that medical laser technologies are nothing more or less than focused energies—and they have made many surgeries minimally invasive, and there are hundreds of applications for stimulating healing using lasers, as well.)

Music is entirely powerful. Michael Tyrrell wrote the series of seven 22:22 masterpieces I mentioned before, called *Wholetones*, and it's an amazing complement to your high-vibration life because he literally wrote them around the harmonics in the most healing frequencies, not the 440 Hz music we have all become accustomed to. He calls for a musical revolution to advance health and peace, beginning with musicians retuning their instruments toward that end.

(Tyrrell also explains that he used as much acoustic music as possible in these miraculous recordings because digital music does not have the vibrational purity of old records and analog recordings, and it has become the modern standard only due to its volume capacity and convenience in data storage and transfer.)

He also wrote a book about healing tones, called *The Sound of Healing*, about frequencies and music, and I've linked you to both the *Wholetones* musical pieces and the book on your Resources page with a discount Michael Tyrrell offers you.

The Frequencies of Words

Words are frequencies, just as sound, light, and substances are. They carry a charge and they have the power to uplift spirits, destroy self-esteem, unite an army, or cause a riot.

Sometimes our words are ill-considered because we are fueled by anger or exhaustion, and we may say words that will forever ring in the head of someone we care about. Lately, a popular phrase when we see a shocking image on Facebook is "I can't unsee that!" I would propose to you, with regard to the effect on the future of our words today, that this is also the case too often:

"You can't unsay that."

You've said things you wish you hadn't. Me too! As we commit to living in high frequencies, we're more measured with the looks we give others, the way we use our words, and even things no one will ever know about, such as whether we let someone in front of us in traffic or give our money to charitable causes.

We know now that karma has scientific underpinning: we are putting out vibrations that stir the energies of the universe, and we can make them better or worse, high-pitched and cacophonic or peaceful and healing.

Whoever taught their child "Sticks and stones may break my bones, but words can never hurt me" is callous indeed, for words can be so devastatingly hurtful that every one of us remembers some particular sentence for thirty or fifty years.

As a competitive tennis player, I recently got my first opportunity ever to attend the US Open. I am always cognizant at pro tennis events of the young preteens who pop up from the sideline to fetch a ball at lightning speed and then get out of the way or to run a towel to the pros between serves. They must be very quick to react and poised on their toes in a crouch, potentially for hours. They always strike me as very serious about this coveted-by-children but unglamorous job.

Occasionally you see a pro bark at one of the young volunteers, speaking harsh words because he didn't move quickly enough or give him the towel he wanted. While I am sure playing in the finals of the US Open is an intense experience, the child—obviously a tennis fan—will remember those words from his idol for the rest of his life. Whether they are words of praise and gratitude or harsh words of criticism, he will remember and internalize them.

It costs us so little to offer words of healing, encouragement, and love to others. And yet they are in short supply in a world fraught with dangerous, critical, angry, tension-filled words, particularly in the anonymity of the Internet.

It's easy to allow ourselves into the vibrations of conflict and strife. Why? Because it's easy to stray mindlessly, surfing the Web or watching the television, where frequencies are so often low and cacophonous—but every moment affects our well-being.

Commitment to living a high-vibration life is equally a commitment to raising the vibration of others around us with our acts of service and our use of words.

In Masaru Emoto's book *The Hidden Messages in Water*, he proves the power of the vibrations of words, capturing what happens to a droplet of water in the process of freezing under a microscope as words are spoken. Words such as *God, forgiveness, love,* and *peace* had the effect of the water freezing into beautiful crystals unique to each word.

But when Emoto spoke negatively charged words such as *evil, you fool, you disgust me, Satan, chaos,* and *death,* noncrystalline, disfigured, broken structures appeared under the microscope as the water froze. Words carry charge!

One of the simplest acts we can perform as we become more mindful of living a higher-vibration existence is to take note of the words we use and shift them toward softer, more loving, more peaceful, more authentically kind words. Randomly tossing off "You look pretty today" to people isn't precisely what I mean. Most of us are good at these somewhat trite gestures, and they aren't significantly meaningful to anyone. What's truly powerful is something genuine, specific, and well-considered that the person in your energy field experiences as "She really sees me."

For instance, you might say something as specific as: "I notice how you treat waitresses, and I think you're as beautiful inside as you are outside, because you do kind things even when no one's watching." If someone said this to you, would you remember it?

We are no different than we were as children: we want to know that we are enough, that we are loved, that we are respected, that we did something well. How you speak to yourself, and about yourself, is a great place to start. *Self-love* is a popular concept currently, and it may seem strange when the world needs less narcissism and more service and generosity. But until we learn to speak kindly to ourselves and think kindly toward ourselves, it's unlikely we'll be particularly helpful or convincing with our words toward others.

If you are a parent, you have likely often considered that your children are not their mistakes. They are better than that, and we see the good in them, the potential in them. Unless we are deeply unhappy parents mired in our own negative issues, we likely don't berate and abuse our children for mistakes they make. But do we abuse and berate ourselves? (If so, our children are watching and in learning how to speak to themselves—kindly and forgivingly, or critically and hatefully.)

Remember we discussed earlier that Deepak Chopra says that the vast majority of our self-talk is negative and critical. Even worse, 95 percent of the negative things we say to ourselves we've said over and over, for days, months, and decades.

I certainly don't want my life to be *Groundhog Day*, do you? Different day, same terrible self-criticism of my body, my abilities, my mistakes.

That's as boring as it is destructive.

I hope you'll commit to being gentle with yourself. Become cognizant of the way you talk to yourself, and talk to yourself as you would to a child you love very much.

Also, let's get back to the Law of Attraction, which is so infused with vibrational science. If you say words such as "My car is a piece of crap, always breaking down," notice how your car breaks down time and again. If you say, "I never win anything," you're actually statistically far less likely to win anything in the company raffle.

If "I don't have time for this" slips from your lips every day, you're likely to find that you're always rushed, always behind, and unproductive. If you say, "I don't have good luck with men," don't expect your dating life to improve!

You may assume that things are often awry in your life because you're unlucky. What if things keep going awry because you expect them to, you verbalize that expectation, and you transmit energies in every way that brings hardship to you?

Words are powerful—and they are easy. They are easy to use thoughtlessly in harmful ways, and easy to use to uplift and inspire. So, less of the former, and more of the latter! Words are a perfect place to start in your experiments with raising your own ViQ—which has the inevitable, exciting effect of raising others' frequency as well!

Accountability, Conscious Compassion, and Random Acts of Kindness

My favorite source for leveraging the divine spark in all of us, in our relationships and in our professions, is found in the works of Terry Warner, PhD, and the Arbinger Institute that he founded.

The three works I can't recommend highly enough are by Warner and his colleagues: *Bonds that Make Us Free, The Anatomy of Peace,* and *Leadership and Self-Deception.* The first title is geared toward your most intimate relationships, the last title is for the workplace, and the middle one is a bit of both.

When *Bonds that Make Us Free* was still just a manuscript on copy paper, I went to a class by a psychologist disciple of Warner's and read the book cover to cover multiple times, and it changed my life as almost no other book ever has. In fact, I am positive that the book you are now reading would not exist if it were not for the influence of Terry Warner and the Arbinger Institute on my work and my life.

It caused me to take full responsibility for my choices, my words, my reactions to events in daily life. These books unflinchingly require the reader to stop blaming others and look in the mirror. I think and act differently as a result of studying Warner's great works.

I read Nietzsche, the nihilists, and many negative assumptions about human nature in my formal studies of philosophy, human psychology, and the art and science of psychotherapy. But nowhere did I read work assuming divine, positive intent by human beings as I did in the Arbinger Institute's works.

I agree with Warner that at our heart center we are compassionate and we want to serve; it is life experiences and negative programming that get in our way. We feel the literal, energetic pull of "doing the right thing" every day toward one another—loved ones and strangers alike—and we become our most authentic selves when we heed the call rather than engaging in acts Warner calls, in all three of the books referenced above, "self-betrayal."

A tremendous amount of energy is lost when we find others to blame or make excuses for our mistakes and the ways we wrong others. When we quickly own responsibility, regardless of complicating circumstances, it drains the negative energy from the situation, and our relationships return to equilibrium quickly because of far less resistance.

Performing acts of service, especially anonymous ones, is part and parcel of adopting the frequencies of compassion. The energetic interpretation of the law of karma is that as you participate in the powerful flow of good works, you increase in compassion and high vibrations. As Ecclesiastes 11:1 in the Bible says, "Cast your bread upon the waters, and after many days it will come back to you."

After one of the most devastating events of my life, I learned to let go, which has been one of the most important ways I've recovered and achieved the highest ViQ of my life in the wake of many challenges. In fact, I sometimes can't believe how much I've changed and how much I let go of now.

Even fifteen to twenty years ago, as a mother of several young children trying to control outcomes with an iron fist, I could not have wrapped my brain around how much "going with the flow" or floating downstream I would become capable of. In fact, it would not have seemed like a good thing at that time. But it is, because we truly cannot control the actions of others, only our reactions to them. I've become far happier and more emotionally healthy by releasing judgments of others' choices.

Prayer and Faith

People of faith are happier people. Whether you're an evangelical Christian, a Hindu, a Jew, a Muslim, a Catholic, an agnostic, or an atheist, believing in something greater than yourself, something powerful and good, makes you healthier. ("Faith" doesn't imply belief in a specific deity; of course, people all over the world look to emulate different deities who have similar attributes. In fact, one can have faith without believing in a system of gods.)

This much is documented in the scientific literature about faith and the power of prayer: we are happier when we believe in something bigger than ourselves and when we have purpose.

And "spiritual" people don't have to be religious to enjoy the benefits. I've gone twice to a Hindu ashram in Texas to study and purify my mind and heart with Eastern spiritual guides (Jain monks and nuns), even though I do not consider myself a member of their religion or community. The idea was to study my own soul and its purpose and how I am treating others. For example, I asked myself during a twelve-day water fast there: Am I committing any acts of violence in the way I treat myself or any other living things? Are my actions in alignment with my beliefs?

Part of why the religious and spiritual tend to say they are happier is the sense of community, purpose, and sharing of a common belief system. And even though the language of religion can sometimes cut both ways, in most religions, punishment, sin, and judgment seem to serve mainly as a counterpoint to the greater feelings of love, hope, and belief in something better and bigger than ourselves.

And it's not only people who are members of an organized religion who experience this. Even those who believe in a higher power and/or profess to be spiritual but don't attend a church, temple, synagogue, or mosque worship in nature or simply wherever they are in an internal way through meditation, prayer, or other spiritual or personal rites and practices. People of every faith report "feeling the Spirit," regardless of how they precisely define that Spirit.

Whatever you believe, I hope you're open to the unknowable. Remember that quantum theory and research show us that almost anything can happen—and does. Study and intellectual pursuits are easy for me. But intuition, wonder, awe, and accepting that many things are unknowable can result in a surrender that is peaceful and transcendent, and letting go and embracing these qualities have made me far happier.

This openness and surrender has the power to raise your ViQ and help others to a higher place as well.

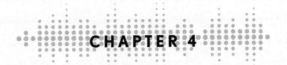

CHAPTER 4

Practices that Lower Vibration

THINGS THAT LOWER

• Stress/Distress: The Kind You Can't or Don't Solve

• Dead, Denatured Foods

• Negative or Toxic People & Relationships

• Being Angry, Fearful, or Depressed

• Inauthenticity, Lying/Cheating/Lack of Integrity

• Resisting Change, Others' Choices, or Consequences of Actions

• Electromagnetic Frequencies (EMFs) from Electronic Devices

Many people think that having a lot of things to do or having a challenging project that they feel anxious about completing on time qualifies as "stress" that is bad for you. In fact, this is a type of stress that can actually be very good for you, according to research. As Dr. Richard Shelton, vice chair for research in the department of psychiatry at the University of Alabama–Birmingham, notes, it's only when stress becomes chronic that it negatively affects our health and well-being. He shares five ways in which a little short-term anxiety can benefit both your body and your brain:

1. Helps boost brainpower by stimulating the production of neurotrophins and strengthening the connections between neurons and the brain.

2. Increases short-term immunity. The body responds to stress by preparing itself for possible infection or injury, and it does this by producing extra interleukins, which help regulate the immune system.

3. Makes you more resilient as you learn to deal with stressful situations, making future ones easier to manage. This also helps you develop a psychological and physical sense of control.

4. Motivates you to succeed. Such things as deadlines stimulate your behavior to manage the situation more rapidly, productively, and effectively. But you must look at such a situation as a doable challenge rather than an impossible roadblock.

5. Can benefit an unborn child. A little stress during a woman's pregnancy can help increase her child's motor and developmental skills by age two.

People need challenges and reasons to get up in the morning. Goals, deadlines, very difficult work, and even a significant amount of pressure can exercise parts of your brain that literally keep you smart and keep you young!

Folks with Alzheimer's and forms of dementia are far more likely than the general population to have spent their spare time watching TV, small-talking, or doing other low-vibration, unchallenging activities. Doing crossword puzzles or Sudoku, reading books on challenging subjects, attending lectures and conferences, painting or playing tennis or engaging in any hobby that uses your brain, continuing your career well past retirement age—these are all great ways to avoid mental decline.

We think of work as something we need a vacation from. However, one of the highest forms of self-actualization, in the pursuit of your Optimal ViQ, is meaningful work.

The kind of stress that makes you sick is "distress," not challenges and deadlines and a healthy amount of pressure. Often, people think that "more vacation" is the way to avoid the negative health effects of stress. While overwork is something we may need breaks from, most of the people of the world get little or no vacation at all, while reporting much higher levels of happiness than Americans do, who vacation a lot.

Negative stress involves chronic situations that cause dread, fear, anxiety, or depression, those that you are not solving or cannot solve.

Examples of "bad" stress are a toxic marriage or other relationship, or employment where you are being undervalued, overworked, or even abused. "Distress" may include working in a war zone, being socially isolated or neglected, having a career you dislike or have little aptitude for, chronic rejection in a social setting you cannot escape, or being in a religious or cultural atmosphere where you are disapproved of.

I very much hope that you will do what it takes to solve any chronic-stress issue in your life—you can drink green juice and do yoga all day, but if you walk in the door every night to an unsolvable problem that ties your stomach in knots, there's going to be a ceiling on what you can accomplish in your upleveling.

Getting space and freedom from two different relationships in my first fifty years was absolutely foundational to being able to write fifteen books, start a multimillion-dollar business, and accomplish many other goals as a sole-custody single mother the past nine years.

I paid dearly for the freedom from these two individuals, but setting boundaries and getting away from two different situations that felt unsolvable to me after many years of effort is something that absolutely must be addressed in any discussion of optimizing my ViQ that I am committed to now.

Dead, Denatured Foods

Living foods, like the green smoothie or green juice I'm encouraging you to start making and drinking every day, are packed with enzymes. Enzymes are a catalyst in all metabolic processes in your body, and you probably remember from high school science classes that they are "used up" in the process. Digestive enzymes are produced primarily by your pancreas but also by your liver, and your body has a finite capacity to produce them.

Unfortunately, because most of what people eat in this age of processed and packaged foods is dead and stripped of its nutrition, we are heavily drawing on those limited enzyme factories in the body. So when we eat all cooked food, we're heavily taxing the body, and the result is organ burnout.

We are living in a social experiment never before attempted, wherein most or all of the diet of most Americans is cooked, and much of it is processed, with the most nutritious or high-fiber parts missing—like the bran (fiber) and germ (vitamins) in the grain, when you eat white-flour baked goods. Like the vitamins and minerals and enzymes destroyed in canned fruits or juices versus the whole food.

Chewing on a piece of sugarcane now and then wouldn't be so terrible, but stripping it of all its fiber and concentrating the sugars is to literally feed the body chemicals that cause haywire reactions.

Eating far more living, raw plant foods is absolutely key to raising your vibration. There is no substitute. There is no pill, no matter how "natural," that can replace the synergistic magic of brightly colored whole plant foods in their complete and authentic package.

In addition to the emotional metabolism we discussed, this is the other "most important" thing to do in the quest we're working on together in this book. Ditch the truly low-value foods, such as products made with white flour, processed meats like hot dogs and bacon, soda of any kind, concentrated sugars, and especially refined sugars—worst of all, corn syrup.

Even worse are the "foods" that aren't really food, the chemical sweeteners like aspartame and Splenda and saccharin, as well as the neurotoxin MSG, ubiquitous in the food supply and hiding in many ingredients and products.

I feel so strongly about it that I've created a wallet card you can print out so you never buy a neurotoxic ingredient again. These ingredients cause migraines and vertigo and damage the brain and myelin sheaths over time, which may lead to high risk of multiple sclerosis, ALS, dementia, Parkinson's, and other degenerative neurological diseases.

I've also given you a GMO wallet card listing the commonly genetically modified foods and ingredients to avoid as well. Print them and put them in your wallet. As we all get educated about GMO foods and stop buying them, they will be driven out of our food system. You can get both cards on your Resources page.

Those are the worst of the bad in vibration-wrecking ingredients and foods. But really, eliminating anything from a fast-food restaurant and 95 percent of what is sold in cans and boxes is a great idea too, if you're willing to go the distance for your health. If it's cheap and/or from a fast-food restaurant, it's highly likely to contain genetically modified, processed foods and worse—chemical additives that are harmful to your vibration.

If any of those foods makes a significant appearance in your regular diet, you'll want to consider that they are almost certainly dragging your ViQ lower.

So what should you eat to achieve high vibrations?

Lots of big, green salads full of colorful vegetables, with some spiced kidney or garbanzo beans or lentils on top. Or if you prefer to drink your veggies, a big green smoothie or juiced greens and root vegetables is the best thing you can do to raise your vibe today, tomorrow, and every single day. This maximizes your nutrition most easily. And if you order green juice from a local juice store, get it fresh and have them leave out the fruit—just greens and veggies. (I promise, if you give this time, you'll love the taste. A little lemon juice and ginger make it so lovely.)

A piece of any fruit you like or a handful of nuts for a snack is another easy, high-vibe habit.

So is decreasing your consumption of animal flesh and dairy products—and make sure any of those you do eat are wild-caught, organic, or free-range (i.e., clean, or cleaner than the processed and conventionally raised meats).

If you undertake the 7-Day Detox at the end of this book, you'll see a powerful cleansing, with all of the good and none of the bad. This exciting experiment may just commit you for life to seeking out far more of the good stuff.

Negative or Toxic People or Relationships

Remember that every time you talk to someone, you're exchanging energies. Your words, and also your body language and your many other ways of communicating, are transmitting subtle energies that profoundly affect whomever you are talking to.

Shouting, swearing, and abusive language harm your energies quickly. When you're the doer of those actions, you're also far more likely to be the receiver of them! Sometimes the problem is with the relationship—the dynamic between two people trapped in a pattern of communication or behavior that neither likes, but they haven't done the work of disentangling those patterns and rebuilding better ones.

But sometimes it's the person you share space with. Perhaps he was raised in a terrifying and unsafe environment, and he learned some coping mechanisms that aren't serving him in his relationship with you.

It's also possible he has a diagnosable personality disorder or mental health issue that gets in the way of a more authentic and loving way of interacting with others. (This is likely to be the case when he repeatedly has the same problems in other relationships that you are experiencing with him.)

And long-term chemical exposure, drug abuse, or a traumatic brain injury can change a person's personality and harm his brain, even eat holes in it—and that can show up as behavioral and emotional disturbance that affects relationships.

This is a difficult topic to discuss, because casting people aside is not something Jesus, or Gandhi, or Mother Teresa would do. That said, I've watched people close to me and people in therapy work with a drug-addicted sister or child for many years, and they all eventually come to the conclusion that they have to have boundaries; they need to protect their own families, property, money, and energies; and they are not bad people if they set limits.

If you haven't given yourself permission to sidestep energy vampires in your life, may I give you permission to do so?

I was raised in a family where, for many generations, marriages were difficult but always stayed together because all parties were deeply committed to the idea of marriage. And I am officially the only divorcée of the eight children in my family, with all the rest married.

For a time, I felt the need to defend my decision to end my twenty-year marriage. After all, he wasn't a porn addict, he wasn't a drug addict, he was a good provider, and he didn't cheat on me or hit me.

As Amy Poehler said in her memoir recently, about the end of her marriage to the actor Will Arnett, "I don't consider a ten-year marriage a failure."

What a brilliant thought. I'm happy that I had the experience of being married and of working out difficult things for many years—and I love the four beautiful children that came from that twenty-year marriage. And I do not consider it a failure. Others felt differently at the time of my divorce, and that is their prerogative. But, as the saying goes, how they feel about me and my choices is none of my business.

When news of our divorce broke, our episode of *Wife Swap* had just aired on ABC, so we were already the talk of the town. But I knew that if I would just lie low and say nothing to harm my ex-husband's name, since he had to live in the community too, or say anything that could hurt my children, everyone would move on after a period of curiosity, questions, and gossip.

And move on they did. There's always new news tomorrow.

Being peaceful with change in relationships is key to health and happiness too. I'm not suggesting that marriage isn't an important commitment. I'm suggesting that we do survive when relationships end, and that as we live at higher frequencies, a natural consequence is that some relationships will die a natural death. As we release them in a peaceful way and accept that things have a life cycle, we embrace the whole of the experience. We achieve more peace, because most relationships are not lifelong, and that does not mean they don't have value and meaning.

There is happiness and growth after the end of a relationship that no longer serves (or never did), and there have to be limits to the energies that an unhealthy relationship in our life is allowed to consume.

Being Anxious or Depressed

These are states of consciousness that are entirely at odds with your health and happiness vibe. In fact, you *cannot* be happy or at peace while experiencing one of these negative emotions. That's why when you feel the emotion of anger, for instance, and identify it as such, you absolutely must Metabolize/Reframe/Release it, as you learned earlier in this book. And because you cannot be happy while experiencing anger or fear, you will get very serious about this process when you realize that anger as a chronic state is not serving you and is actually hurting you.

Telling others about it doesn't always "get it off your chest," and, in fact, often that venting of negative energies just incubates the negative feelings—plus, it harms the person you're telling about it, the unlucky listener who is now trapped in those energies.

It does nothing to resolve the situation between you and whomever you are angry with, and hurts you far, far more than it hurts whoever has wronged you. Anger has an important function, to mobilize us toward action. But as a chronic state of being, it doesn't have any utility except to make us miserable.

Fear is an emotion that bears discussion, since 25 percent of Americans now report having significant anxiety. Millions of pills are taken to mitigate the chronic fear affecting quality of life for a quarter of us every single day. My theory is that as thousands of chemicals are in active use in our food, air, and water every day, hormone disruptors cause daily misfires for millions of us, and anxiety is a common result. (*Anxiety* is the clinical word, but the emotion is fear.)

But that's not all of my theory. The other part of it involves the changed media environment we're exposed to and the headlong rate of change that technology imposes on virtually everyone in any professional environment.

We often hear that technology makes life better. But the more technologies proliferate, the faster the speed of change in business is as your competitors use the new app, the new system, the new software to excel in your field of work. So, in essence, you are forced to change or die.

My son and I had a funny conversation the week he turned sixteen about how he turns the steering wheel in my car so far to the right or left that it hits its limit. As I taught him how to drive, I often reminded him, "When you feel it hit like that? You've gone too far."

When I said that to him last year, he retorted, "I hate driving your car."

I replied, astonished, "You *hate* driving a Lexus?"

He replied, "Well, it's just so touchy, compared to my Corolla."

Now, Tennyson's Corolla is eight years old, and, ironically, his friend Spencer calls the Corolla "touchy"—because Spencer was gifted his grandpa's 1993 Ford pickup truck. Ah, the lesson in how everything is relative.

Tennyson was very excited about my trading the Lexus in for a new Tesla S recently and was lobbying to get to drive it to homecoming. I said, "Well, if you think the Lexus is touchy, just wait till we get the Tesla."

It goes from 0 to 60 in 3.5 seconds.

Grandpa's 1993 Ford pickup truck, Tennyson's 2008 Toyota Corolla, my 2013 Lexus, my hot-off-the-line Tesla S. This feels like a metaphor of how life has been accelerating in the past decade—the most rapid decade of growth in the history of mankind. Touchier and touchier.

And you're living it.

No wonder we're all an anxious mess. Who wouldn't be? Nothing in our biology or history has prepared us for this moment.

Hence my choice to write this book about ways I've discovered to achieve Zen in this fast-paced world and to protect our vibration, even as life gets increasingly chaotic.

I believe that this frenetic pace of change, faster everything, and invisible electrical and magnetic currents in the environment all around us can cause a tremendous amount of anxiety, contributing significantly to what looks like an anxiety epidemic.

We now go faster, are more efficient, and have access to so much data that most professional climates can feel very intense and stressful. My own employees and I discuss this on a regular basis: how breathless we feel, exposed instantaneously to what all of our competitors are doing at the touch of a key because of the Internet, aware of all the things we should be doing but don't have enough hours in the day to learn and implement.

I've completely opted out of watching the news as part of my own strategy to lead a peaceful and centered life in the face of so much chaos and never-ending speed and acceleration.

But I also recommend the grounding practices in this book, to observe the chaos and change in the world and be able to channel it mindfully in your professional work—without losing your mind in the rest of your life.

Falseness: Inauthenticity, Lying, Cheating, Lack of Integrity

Some studies indicate that in the course of any day, you hear quite a shocking number of lies. Because of this, we have all become, to varying degrees, cynical about what we hear and read.

In my teens, I experimented with lying. I was partying with my friends while living in a teetotaling, very strict Mormon home, so my actions were in conflict with my parents' wishes for me. Rather than adhere to their standards, I experimented with drinking and other forms of "breaking the rules" my entire senior year of high school.

The worst part, for me, was lying. An energy healer would say that my energies were going one direction, and my behavior was going the opposite direction. Or that my energies were at odds! It's no wonder I spent most of that year of rebellion, having been a very "good girl" my whole life, with my stomach tied in knots.

It's an important part of our developmental tasks as adults to check in with ourselves on a daily basis by asking this:

Are my words and actions authentic and in harmony with each other?

If I feel discomfort with how I am presenting myself, what is it that's bothering me?

Anyone with a deep desire to live authentically knows that truth telling is absolutely imperative in that goal. Not that you have to be brutal or even direct when asked, "Honey, does this dress make me look fat?"

We could debate whether there are times to fudge the truth. But let's talk about the straightforward 99 percent of the time, when our words and the truth are incongruous, which decreases our integrity and, therefore, our ability to achieve optimal ViQ.

Usually, if we're posing in any social environment, it comes from a desire for someone to like us—and our sense that they won't if they know the limits of our abilities or accomplishments.

At some point, probably after years of practicing checking in with yourself, you may become keenly aware of your insecurities and gently call yourself out on them. You may be willing, then, to practice being true to exactly who you really are.

And if you do, you discover a marvelous truth: that people actually like you better when you're nothing more, and nothing less, than who you are. Bragging, lying, posing, and all forms of inauthenticity are easily discernible by intuition, because they come in an energetic package that is undeniable.

Even if people can't put their finger on it, they know they don't like jarring energetics and that they make them uncomfortable. They'll avoid you, they won't do business with you, they won't trust you—and, in the final analysis, that's harmful to you, especially as it becomes a pattern. The Law of Attraction, after all, cuts both ways. Posing and deceit do not attract success and high vibration.

The conclusion? It's always better to just be you. Practice it, because you'll learn that you're lovable regardless of your failings and flaws.

Tell the truth in a job interview that you don't know how to do something.

Speak up at work when you're uncomfortable with the ethics of a marketing campaign.

Admit to doing something mean-spirited, because it clears the air and lets you begin again in a relationship.

I belong to four different influencer networks—places where wellness and personal-growth authors hang out together. We network, we form business alliances, and we listen to content from the stage about various subjects that affect all of us who are running businesses online. We go out for cocktails afterward, and that's where things get real. Those willing to be authentic will discuss our struggles and failures and challenges, in the hopes that our peers have something to offer: words of advice or connections to folks who might help us solve our issues.

Being in these communities is exciting, because there's a lot of powerful energy with so much IQ, so many accomplishments, dozens of *New York Times* bestselling authors in every room I've ever been in with this crowd. Frequently, attendees refer to feeling "intimidated"—and even though I believe we all put our pants on one leg at a time, and it's a core value of mine to lean into my fears, I still can relate.

It's been a game changer for me to come out of the online corner I worked in all by myself for many years and join these networks. But recently I had an interesting experience when one of the events I attended featured a highly controversial speaker.

Without being too specific, I'll tell you that he was only forty, a new network television show was airing based on his extraordinary life, he claimed to have founded multiple billion-dollar companies, and he asserted that he had one of the highest IQs of all the human beings alive today who have taken the test. And he had stories of intrigue and working with high-level governments to save lives. It was all rather spectacular!

As he shared his story and talked about what one of his purported fourteen companies does, the very environment in the room became highly charged. Finally, another CEO piped up and asked, rather provocatively, "There are lots of negative things about you on the Internet, in the media—are you for real? I've got to say, some of what you say seems unbelievable."

Afterward, this man and his story were the subject of many heated private conversations, and I noted with interest how negatively many of the other business owners felt about his story. "I don't believe any of it" was a common theme.

I don't have any agenda judging his story, which may be 100 percent true, for all I know. What is interesting here is the big, palpable reaction of others to this man's grand tale (true or not).

We all crave authenticity and connection in this world where we're constantly bombarded with information and so much of life is moving onto a medium called the Internet.

It's no longer hard to find information. Nobody knows what the Dewey Decimal System is anymore. (It's an organizational concept for libraries that those of us old enough to have grown up pre-Internet had to learn.) Information is everywhere and can be obtained in seconds. But now we're left with a new challenge: What's true? How do I sift through all this information?

Most of the "information" on the Internet now is marketing. It was written with an agenda, using cherry-picked "facts," by professional writers trained in persuasive copywriting. Even a non-selling message has an agenda of getting you to "opt in" so you can be marketed to later. So even what doesn't seem to be marketing actually is.

What I get from my readers now, which is completely different than in 2007 when I put up GreenSmoothieGirl.com, is "Hey, GSG, I read thus-and-such. Is it true?"

So, finding information is no longer a challenge, but we're all fine-tuning our discernment radar as fast as we can as the information avalanche, organized by Google and the other search engines, is now trillions of gigabytes and growing.

Authenticity, integrity, and truth-telling are at an all-time premium. We're overloaded with information, but nobody knows what the truth is anymore.

We don't care how many *New York Times* bestsellers you've written. We don't care how much money you make. We want to know we can believe you, we can trust you, and we are safe with you.

You show us you're a truth teller by having hard conversations with us, where you might say something that could be uncomfortable, maybe even hurtful—but you do it with clarity and love.

You show us you're a truth teller by telling us where you've failed and where you're weak. Brené Brown has brought the message of how powerful it is, in your relationships and your engagement in the world, to be willing to be *vulnerable*.

Then the things you accomplish have rich meaning. You've achieved depth, in our eyes, in a shallow world. We believe what you say next.

Your grandpa would tell you this, and he would be the expert on this, far more than you or I: at the end of your life, you'll die having nothing but your name anyway.

Accomplishment is less impressive than total sincerity is. When you practice always telling the truth, you are in synchronicity with all your energies—which can continue to flow forward rather than getting jumbled, causing you to spend your time and energies remembering and defending half-truths or lies and developing self-justifying stories to try to resolve your own discomfort in the dissonance of your integrity falling apart.

After all, whomever you lied to will walk away and start thinking about something else. You, however, get to sit with that lie or deception forever, until you energetically resolve it.

Asking for forgiveness, making a commitment to act in integrity in all your actions, doing the right thing even though the wrong thing tempts you, being "you" in a very real way rather than someone else you wish you were—these are all examples of cleaning your energies. It will serve you well in your quest for a high-vibration life.

Resisting Change, Others' Actions, or Consequences of Your Actions

Change is inevitable, and those who learn to embrace it win!

In these first fifty years, I've seen such dramatic shifts in the stages of my life that they almost seem to have nothing to do with each other. One of the most important things I've learned is to work hard while simultaneously floating with the current rather than against it.

It's almost as if I've reinvented myself every seven years, as the press says Madonna has.

I bet you have done some reinventing too. One almost has to in order to remain viable and keep up with the pace of change in the modern world.

Then there are the phases of my personal life, the partners I've danced with (married for twenty years, and several serious relationships in the past ten). I have learned that if I stay energetically stuck in a relationship, my growth is slowed.

If I embrace rather than resist each new stage, I'm happier. My adult phases include being a single college student; then married, pursuing a professional career, and working through years of infertility issues with my husband; then a wife and mom, raising four small children born within six years of one another; then a single mom to teens and young adults. Soon I'll be single with kids raised and gone—and little grandchildren, probably.

Happiness means loving and embracing the phase I'm in, learning everything I can from it, and being at peace with the fact that it, like all else, will come to an end.

And why not reinvent and be willing to grow? The more comfortable we are with change, the more adaptable we make ourselves and the more we "roll with the punches" and enjoy life and the neverending variety we encounter.

I've become so adaptable, embracing "new normals," that in some ways I almost worry that I've become too tolerant of change. There's almost nothing that surprises me. "Truth is stranger than fiction" has become a mantra for me as life unfolds.

Every time I reach a new normal, I know that it's just a way station until more upheaval and change that I could not have predicted, and cannot control, come along. Nothing about life has been predictable except for the constant of change!

My entire career has been reborn many times. I've rebuilt from nothing over and over. The half-life of my formal education gets shorter and shorter, with more technologies, more apps, more acceleration from the information age of fifteen years ago to the digital age we've entered.

My kids were babies, toddlers, preteens, teenagers, and now adults. I can't get too attached to the current phase they're in, because they keep "becoming."

But I can enjoy the process and the path. After all, change is inevitable.

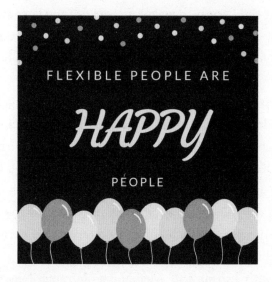

Flexible people are happy people!

Avoiding change or resisting what must be embraced, rather than leaning into the wind, only creates a feeling of being stuck.

Steven Pressfield, in the great classic *The War of Art*, says, "Resistance cannot be seen, touched, heard, or smelled. But it can be felt. We experience it as an energy field radiating from a work-in-potential. It's a repelling force. It's negative. Its aim is to shove us away, distract us, prevent us from doing our work."

Pressfield says that things we resist tend to be any diet or health regimen; any program of spiritual advancement; education; the pursuit of any calling in writing, painting, music, film, dance, etc.; and acts of political, moral, or ethical courage, including the decision to change our thought or conduct. We also tend to resist making a big commitment to another person, taking a principled stand against something we believe to be morally wrong, and undertaking an effort to help others.

In other words, Pressfield says, we create resistance to "any act that rejects immediate gratification in favor of long-term growth, health, or integrity."

I have also found, as a parent, that my resistance to a choice my teen or adult child wants to make can backfire and become a motivator to do exactly the thing I don't want him or her to do. (I'll show Mom who's in charge!) So my useless resistance harms our relationship.

I'm not suggesting that you don't take a stand against something your child wants to do that is not in her best interests. I absolutely do that and will continue to do it. However, I have many times found myself in opposition to a decision that is really, in the scheme of things, a minor issue, not affecting my child's health or integrity or future in a significant way, and my resistance to the choice has harmed my relationship with her. (This is to say, I've learned this lesson the hard way.)

So, as with learning to Metabolize/Reframe/Release negative emotions, I go through a similar process when my child makes a choice I do not like. An example is when Tennyson chose to drop out of his AP classes to take easier ones. I wasn't happy about it, and I made a passionate speech in favor of choosing quality, choosing to be challenged, and rising to the challenge. And then I got out of the way, because he is old enough to make his own choices in this arena. I'm not going to decline any teaching opportunity, because I know that while my kids may roll their eyes and act dismissive, it does sink in. They do want my approval, they want to clear the high bar of my standards—and my words do have an impact, over time.

Another example is Emma's recent trip to Greece, which I briefly mentioned earlier. I'd just given her $5,000 for school expenses after she told me she was struggling to get decent grades while working two jobs.

Suddenly she decided she was going to Greece with a friend for a month during the summer, even though this would be the fourth summer in a row she'd taken an international trip, and my opinion (which her father shared) was that she should be working all summer. As we did, making sacrifices. I felt that adventuring could wait until she'd finished her degree and she had discretionary income.

She pitched me repeatedly on how she had it all worked out to be an extremely inexpensive trip, and I decided, after clearly stating how I felt about it, to avoid letting the situation make a negative impact on our relationship. I bit my tongue for the few months until she left on the trip. During her trip, I enjoyed her daily travelogue and photos, hearing about the people she met and the things she did. I trusted that her coming back with her savings very thin would be a good "life lesson" opportunity for her.

The more I parent young adult children, the more I learn to let go and release them to be who they are, make their mistakes, and learn from them.

I am not suggesting we shouldn't sometimes resist our children's choices. If one of my children started using crystal meth or wanted to drop out of college to be a stripper, I'd resist! I'm simply suggesting that others make choices that affect us almost daily, and we get to choose what we'll do with that. Coming to peace, sooner rather than later, with choices that aren't what we would have made is good for our health—and good for our relationships of love and trust.

We also have a tendency to resist the consequences of our actions. When we accept and submit to some of the things that life deals us— not the injustices and the things we need to speak up about but the natural consequences of our actions—we're happier and more in harmony with the flow of the universe.

A friend of mine, whom I'll call Cinda, has a seventeen-year-old daughter—I'll call her Amie—who was caught driving without a license and with marijuana paraphernalia in her car. Amie was sentenced to do community service hours and did not complete them. The year got away from them, busy with work and school, and when Cinda realized they'd run out of time, she filled out the form for the court to prove Amie had done the community service—and asked her friends, including me, if we would vouch for her daughter's service to our businesses, if the state called us.

The message given to the child here is: "You can dodge the consequences of your actions by lying and cheating, and I'll help you do it."

This doesn't serve Amie well, and it squanders an opportunity for her to learn from the effects of her actions.

One of the great criticisms of the millennial generation is that they are spoiled from being given too much and being shielded from the natural consequences of their choices. These are the kids who were all given trophies after the soccer season, even if they were on the losing team.

How much have you learned from the consequences of failing to study in school, or of procrastinating on a project at work, or of not communicating about a major problem in a relationship? And especially from facing the consequences, which tend to be the world's greatest teachers? How much growth would you have forgone if someone had taken those consequences away, so that you never had to feel any discomfort in your formative years?

One of the most difficult things in parenting, I think, is to love my children enough to let them suffer a bit—sometimes more than a bit—without rescuing them when they are faced with a consequence imposed by the school, the law, or another person in authority.

Electromagnetic Frequencies (EMF) in Your Environment

Never before in history have we had as many as six different electrical devices in our energy field at any given time.

What happens when we have disruptive, chaotic, low, and competing frequencies in our energy field? No one is entirely sure—but ten to twenty years from now, we'll know with chilling certainty, because plenty of curious researchers are undertaking longitudinal studies.

Some evidence shows breast cancers in the exact shape of cell phones that were put inside a bra, many hours a day, for years. And brain tumors the shape of, and in the exact location of, cell phones held to the ear. By 1971, the U.S. Naval Research Laboratory had collected almost 1,800 studies on the effects on humans of EMF, or electromagnetic frequencies. Since then, more than 8,000 more studies have been published.

Evidence is fast emerging that the human organism's sensitive frequencies are interrupted by the "chaotic" frequencies of cell phones, microwaves, computers, iPads—even pencil sharpeners!

I'm concerned about the experiment of our children having these radioactive wavelengths in their force fields almost twenty-four hours a day—the first generation ever of children exposed to so many disordered frequencies every day.

Could it be related to the epidemic of attention deficit disorder (ADD), as some hypothesize? With increasing numbers of toxic vaccines, medications, and genetically modified foods, we've got many contenders in the theories about what's causing the rise in ADD (and ADHD).

I know people so committed to reducing their EMF exposure that they turn off the electricity at the source, on the power grid, every night before bed. Apparently, the freezer and fridge keep things cold enough all night long.

This is likely taking the issue further than most of us are willing to. For the rest of us, there are some easy practices for grounding and strengthening the nervous system and raising our vibration. On your Resources page, I've provided an EMF Action Plan that covers ways you can protect yourself from EMF frequencies in your home and at work, including easy and free or inexpensive solutions to start with. When I measured the "dirty electricity" in my home and installed filters on each outlet that measured high, I slept through the night, and the next three nights, for the first time in twenty years!

Our whole agenda in this book is "getting high" without the negative consequences to the nervous system of substance-induced highs. What we're learning here are sustainable practices for a lifetime, with countless health benefits.

Remember, it's not simply an increased amplitude of frequency or higher waves per second that we want—it's also cohesive frequencies. We want harmonic vibrations, such as you get when you hit a tuning fork—not the chaotic, random frequencies of the wires strung from telephone poles to carry bits of data, and the phone in your pocket, and the laptop in front of you. Those are all emitting various wavelengths, including radioactive frequencies.

These messy vibrations harm our own harmonic, our strong vibrations, and, consequently, our physical and emotional health.

You may have read about how some scientists think that chaotic frequencies from cell phone towers, telephone wires, and all the EMF hovering above earth may be what's adversely affecting the honeybee population of the world: disorienting them, lowering their honey production, making them more aggressive, and even sometimes killing them. But some studies go further, suggesting that these frequencies also adversely affect other insects, birds, and other animals—and also plants!

Although, in general, higher is better with frequencies, grounding is also a part of our goal, to both increase symbiotic electric energy and make it uniform, predictable, and tranquil.

Obviously, we don't want the high, creative frequencies when we're in the theta stage of sleep. A low, restorative frequency is entirely appropriate then—but still calm and grounded, for peaceful, uninterrupted rest.

That's in stark contrast to the random competing frequencies of the mass of electronics in our space when we have five devices plugged in or operating wirelessly in our energy field!

Whatever you do during the day, at a minimum, get all electronics out of your space while you sleep. And follow some simple and easy practices I've shared with you in the EMF Action Plan.

Can We Talk about Your Electronics Addiction?

Let's talk about electronics addiction, which is harmful on a variety of levels besides your vibration. Of course we need our devices to engage in the modern world. But let me ask you a question:

How long could you go without using your devices or electronics?

Let's talk about addiction, social withdrawal, fragmented focus, and just general time kill.

If you're feeling twitchy after just twenty minutes of being deprived of your phone; if it feels like missing limb syndrome (what an amputee feels, for years); if your mind is coming unglued wondering what you're missing online—you're not alone. You're an addict. And the following will surprise you.

Data says that electronics addiction is just as prevalent among older adults, who didn't start adulthood in the digital age, as it is among teenagers! The average American between the ages of eighteen and sixty-four spends more than three hours just on social media per day—then add in the time spent surfing the Internet, gaming, online gambling, texting, etc. Technology addiction is an actual medical/psychological disorder, and there are even doctors, clinics, and (ironically) websites that specialize in treating it as one would treat drug or alcohol addiction.

Of course you're not fully present with the people you care about—your family, your coworkers, your lover—if you're obsessed with the little six-inch gadget in your pocket. This addiction is subtly harmful to your relationships.

I wonder how many times people sitting in a restaurant have been annoyed with their companions because they keep checking their phones. (Millions of times, would you guess?)

One summer, my children and I drove up the canyon near our home or went out to dinner every Sunday, and I made a highly resisted rule that everyone had to leave their cell phones in a bowl on the kitchen counter—me included. You would have thought I was trying to separate them from a kidney.

I dated a guy right after my divorce ten years ago, and we had a brief relationship in which we'd fly back and forth between San Diego, where he lives, and Salt Lake City, where I live.

I moved on to a long relationship with someone local. But when my relationship with the San Diego friend ended, he spent five years trying to convince me to see him again. Finally, when he was in town visiting his twin boys one winter, I agreed to meet him for dinner.

I knew he described himself as ADHD, but when he never put his phone away through the entire dinner, and I saw him a few times looking not at texts in case his kids had an emergency but at Facebook, I had these thoughts:

"Why did I drive all the way up here for this? He's on a date with Facebook. I'm an accessory. I think I'll not do this ever again."

And, as with so many things in life, he never knew that's why I wouldn't get together with him again during his extended visit to Utah that winter. (Or ever.)

Just like I don't write back to every job applicant who wants me to hire them to tell them their inability to use the English language functionally cost them an interview.

We never learn from so many of our losses in life because we didn't get the feedback. But I'm letting *you* in on that little secret.

My former lover may not know why I blew him off. But this lesson remains:

We have so many uphill battles in the effort to find friends or lovers we can really commit to and spend our precious time with.

Our inability to authentically connect with them shouldn't be compounded by something as ridiculous as an addiction to a phone.

Like millions of other diners in Everywhere, USA (and the whole world, in fact), I felt really uninteresting, jilted, and slightly bored while I had dinner with someone on a date with his phone.

Ironically, my hero Nikola Tesla—while generating extraordinary ideas his entire life that led to harnessing the power of Niagara Falls, designing the alternating curent (AC) electrical system, and acquiring about three hundred patents globally—was your typical introverted mad scientist.

He was attractive to women, and they tried to chase him. Beautiful, famous women.

But he may have been the first person on the planet with the social withdrawal symptoms of electrical gadgetry addiction.

He stated that he destroyed his own sexuality at the age of forty. (No one is sure what that means.) He didn't know what to do with his sexuality—it interfered with his scientific goals—and he became more and more reclusive and never was in an intimate relationship of any significance.

In his seventies, after being injured by a taxi, he lived his final years in a New York City hotel room, where his hobby was rehabilitating wounded pigeons.

My theory is that the pigeons were his contact with living creatures, his surrogate. Since he never mastered human contact or enjoyed that extraordinary electron exchange of two human beings in synchronicity, he found a way to meet those needs through other living beings.

Well, why not? Tesla's way might be different than most of ours, as we need and want contact with people.

But—how magical is discussing ideas, when yours plus mine become more than the sum of the parts? Listening to and savoring the unique experience and perspective of someone who is older than you, who grew up in another era, perhaps on another continent.

How valuable is looking into another person's eyes, which doesn't have to be sexual—that electrical feeling when you look into the eyes of someone you've just met and resonate with? The pulse of discovery.

These are all energetic exchange, they're all powerful, and no electronic device can replace the wavelengths of experience with animals and humans.

Devices and social media are adulterated forms of contact that leave us vaguely dissatisfied, buzzing with disjointed frequencies rather than the long and strong vibe of, for instance, a conversation with someone you trust and love.

Let's use the example of me writing this book. Steven Pressman says, in *The War of Art*, that what writers know, and wannabe writers don't, is that it's not writing the book that's hard. It's sitting down to write the book.

I'll use a writing project as an example, since I'm writing to you right now:

When you go on a social media and electronics diet, you are capable of using your entire brain and producing a high-quality piece of communication when, for example, you aren't interrupted once during each paragraph.

When I do a task while talking on the phone, I'm able to operate from only one piece of my brain at a time, which means a lower-quality conversation or lower-quality work.

I need my entire brain to write well, and being interrupted by pinging text messages does not serve that end.

Plus, when you foster and seek that state of deeply immersed flow that enhances any activity you stay focused on for a few hours, your brain makes connections more seamlessly, you express yourself more effortlessly and without stress, and you enjoy your work more.

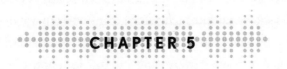

CHAPTER 5

Substances That Raise (and Lower) Vibration

n this chapter, we'll explore the application of the fourth principle from the introduction: "A substance with a higher frequency can cause the vibration of a substance with a lower frequency to increase."

The converse, of course, is true as well. Substances with a low vibration will lower your own frequencies just by being in your energy field, but even more so if you apply them to your skin or consume them.

Let's examine how you can leverage substances in the environment in your goal to achieve the high-vibration life!

::::: CLEAN, MINERAL-RICH WATER :::::

You probably already know that water is required for electrical conductivity. The human being, as we've established, is an electrical being, and it's no accident that the body is comprised of more than 55 percent water. Not just your blood and lymph and other fluids, but every cell is made of more water than any other material.

It's a critical fluid for electrical conductivity—and it's absolutely fundamental to a high-vibration life as well.

Water is needed to flush toxins every day, and it's the most important resource for your colon, liver, kidneys, lymphatic system, and skin.

Studies show that most of us don't drink enough water—which is, for a 150-pound person, about nine glasses of water a day. You know that you need it to avoid overeating and to "clean house," so to speak. But now consider that you need it for electrical conductivity.

That's right, a fully hydrated person is not only cleaner in many different ways but is also capable of high vibration!

Dr. Gerald Pollack, author of *The Fourth Phase of Water*, discusses the many facets of water that science doesn't understand, positing that vibrations are held in the watery spaces in our cells. He calls this unique phase of the H_2O molecule neither liquid, solid, nor vapor but, rather, "living water" that can hold energy, much like a battery, and deliver energy as well.

One of the most useful things I learned to do, as I turned my health around after being very ill in my twenties, is to drink a pint of water first thing when I wake up. To increase electrical conductivity even more, I add concentrated fulvic and humic acids to my morning water, and another dropperful in my water right before bed. I'll tell you more about that on your Resources page, if you wish to learn more.

But I don't drink tap water, because I don't want to drink the fluoride, chlorine, residual pharmaceuticals, pesticides, and even arsenic, found in most city water. So I use a reverse osmosis filter, and I also use a water ionizer so that my water is alkaline.

I love that with the ionizer I can alter the pH of the water I drink and cook with—it's like the natural, clean spring water that runs over rocks in a place such as the Alps, far away from a city.

As you probably do, I live in a city where giant water tanks must be treated with chemicals to prevent outbreaks of E. coli and other bacterial threats to large populations.

Meantime, our vegetables and greens don't have adequate minerals in them, as they used to. Decades of treatment with pesticides and herbicides—and abandoning the practices of allowing fields to lie fallow, rotating crops, and augmenting the soil using compost—has dramatically decreased the nutrient density of our foods. Crops are propped up with chemical fertilizers sprayed on them, which do not have the ability to produce vegetables and fruits with the levels of vitamins, minerals, and enzymes found in organic crops that are treated traditionally and more naturally.

It's the fulvic and humic acids in that black, decomposed plant matter that provide the needed minerals in plants. The plants need them, but we humans absorb minerals from plants—not from rocks or chalk, which are what most mineral supplements you may be buying are made from.

(The human body doesn't understand rocks or chalk as food or medicine. Rocks and chalk are very high in minerals, but they aren't very "bioavailable" to us. The minerals in plants, however, are.)

I finally found an organic, concentrated, plant-based fulvic and humic acid source deep in the earth in Texas, from ancient plant deposits that have not yet turned to shale. It's also naturally got a lot of vitamins and electrolytes and has countless functions I need for my own optimized ViQ.

Using this one supplement daily in clean, remineralized alkaline water has changed my health as much as making the shift to whole foods and mostly plants did years ago!

By adding a dropperful to my drinking water first thing in the morning and last thing before bed, I solved decades of insomnia and now sleep like a baby. (The neurological system needs trace minerals, in balance, to perform its job. And at 11 p.m., the job of the system is to quiet itself and shut down to rest, rebuild, and repair. Who knew that I couldn't fall asleep, from the age of ten onward, because I was missing some raw materials that my neurological system—which is electrical!—required to work properly?)

I thought I had the equivalent of a PhD in health, wellness, and nutrition after so much study when my toddler son and I became so ill, and I turned it around with knowledge and practical application.

But I learned at the age of forty-two something incredibly powerful that has also helped thousands of others since then—the benefit of adding rich fulvic and humic acids, electrolytes, and other nutrients to my water. It was a serious needle mover and a missing link.

I've lost hundreds of hours of sleep, not knowing the answer was as fundamental as getting the right amounts (and ratios!) of all the minerals and trace minerals found in decaying plants—which, of course, are the food of the soil.

It's unfortunate that our soil is so depleted and that chemicals in our air and water also rob us of minerals, but I feel very blessed to have discovered a solution that absolutely works to compensate.

Using this rich fulvic and humic acid compound, two or three droppers full a day, caused my hair to start growing twice as fast and thicker. My fingernails did the same, and they still grow much faster than they did before. My nails are thick and strong. My occasional and mild adult acne disappeared and never came back, and the dark circles under my eyes also disappeared.

All of these (healthy hair, nails, skin, and neurological system) are functions of minerals. And in fact, every single transaction in the body uses minerals and trace minerals. They're being used up by everything the body does, so we have to keep a steady supply coming in. The only place in nature where every single mineral and all the trace minerals known to man are found is in this deep-earth compound of fulvic and humic acids.

It's been a miracle in my life, this discovery. Replacing the minerals in my water with this perfect source gives my body the conductivity it needs to optimize energy and productivity in the morning and all day, without craving stimulants that cause crashes and depletion later, with the vicious cycle starting over again every day.

If you wish to learn more, see "Minerals" on your Resources page.

:::: DRUGS AND ALCOHOL ::::

The crazy thing about writing this section is that, of course, I'm going to tell you how negative drugs and alcohol are for you on every level, including spiritually. But . . .

If you haven't noticed, this entire book is actually teaching you how to get high!

Think about that for a minute. I totally understand why so many people in the modern world look to stimulants, alcohol, marijuana, psychotropic meds, or street drugs daily: to change how they feel.

After all, that's our number-one objective every day, to feel good at every level of Maslow's famous hierarchy of human needs: from lower-level social belonging to higher-level self-actualization.

So what I'm proposing is that we all want to get high. And there's nothing wrong with that, in principle. But increasing your Vibration Quotient is a powerful, sustainable, healthy thing to do. It involves cleaning your cells, purifying the physical vessel, and enlightening and disciplining the mind. That is a "high" far superior to any other— and while it takes some effort, it's all effort you've been meaning to make anyway. Probably for years.

Sure, numbing out by drinking a whole bottle of Chardonnay in front of the TV is easier. But it's unsustainable—you feel worse in the morning, and you wake up half a pound heavier (again) and feeling miserable. And thus begins the downward spiral.

Are you ready for a new kind of high?

It almost goes without saying that alcohol use lowers vibration. The problem, similar to that with coffee and stimulants (opposite effect, similar rationale for the user), is that it alters your state of being in a way that, during the buzz itself, is altogether pleasant for most people. This causes addiction and a cycle of robbing the body of its higher purpose for a short-term fix.

It's the classic example of stealing from tomorrow for pleasure today, so folks who operate from their limbic brain, or young people with an underdeveloped frontal lobe where consequence-oriented thinking occurs, struggle with "delay of gratification." They're in far more danger of spiraling into a constant low-vibration state with drugs and other substances that actually do brain damage over time, not to mention the well-known liver damage.

If you drink, even if you don't consume enough to "get drunk," you know that the next morning you wake up feeling low. You don't have to be hungover, with a headache and maybe even throwing up, for your decreased vibration to tell you that something—maybe you can't put your finger on it—is off. Most likely, you just don't have a lot of energy, and perhaps you do have a low-grade depressive mood.

This is a great time to examine why you drink, how much you drink, and whether a change in these practices would be worth whatever advantage it has for you. Most drinkers report simply liking social interactions better when under the influence.

Social fear disappears, and most people find themselves more verbal, friendly, and at ease in a group. People who drink tend not to fret about time passing and they don't watch the clock, as they might do all day. They just enjoy being mellow, escaping their day-to-day stress by numbing out with the manufactured feeling of well-being and thinking they're engaging more meaningfully with people at a party.

Of course, taking street drugs, or even legal pharmaceuticals, will "toxify" many of your organs and lower your vibe. And I would not tell you to stop taking a pharmaceutical drug, which would be unethical, since once you've started some drugs, some experts say they must be continued forever (for many years, this was the prevailing thinking about blood thinners after a thrombosis event, for instance).

But some who tune in to their body's health learn about alternatives to drugs and balance their systems, including their vibration, with little or no dependence on chemical drugs.

Both prescribed drugs and street drugs are devastating to the perfectly tuned electrical system of the body, sending many organs scrambling to find equilibrium after the disorder wrought by amphetamines, opiates, and many other medications. (Keep in mind that some amphetamines and opiates are prescribed by doctors, while others can get you sent to prison for using them. It's debatable whether there's truly a health risk distinction between the legal and illegal ones, or if it's all simply related to business and politics and controlled quantities.)

The marijuana debate rages on, about whether it's a sin or a virtue, since pot has become widely regarded as innocuous, at least relatively speaking. Perhaps part of why our culture is more and more friendly to weed is due to how lethal street drugs have become in the past decade or two. Marijuana looks tame in comparison. But marijuana sources have become more potent and hybridized, and pot is often cut with other materials, and is sometimes truly dangerous too.

Cannabis oil, or cannabis in various forms, isolates the medicinal part of the plant, which does not intoxicate. There is growing evidence that this substance from the marijuana plant can be very helpful in pain relief.

Pot smoking is another thing altogether. There is plenty of evidence, accumulated for decades, that smoking marijuana causes slow, long-term brain damage, and it most certainly lowers vibration. It also makes weight gain more likely, since, notoriously, if you're high, you're also hungry! And adding pounds beyond a healthy weight invariably brings your vibration very low.

While it's entirely possible that alcohol is more toxic than marijuana is, that doesn't mean smoking weed is a healthy habit. And, of course, as of this writing, it's also illegal in most states. While I think that is in the process of changing as more citizens lobby for legalizing marijuana, and while for the sake of your health I'd probably choose for you to smoke pot occasionally (if it's legal where you live) versus drinking most alcoholic beverages, it's still something to eliminate if you want your highest possible ViQ!

::::: ESSENTIAL OILS AND HERBS :::::

Herbs—the dried stems, roots, or flowers of medicinal plants—were the gold standard in natural healing for many years until recently, when the properties of essential oils were studied and found to be many times more potent than the dried whole plant.

Herbs are less expensive and available at virtually any natural-products store and online. The one advantage they may have over essential oils is that you don't have to worry about what else is in the formula, besides the one herb or several in a blend.

The essential oil is the very essence of the plant, wherever its highest frequency is—and that is found variously in petals, stems, roots, or other parts of the plant.

More than 98 percent of essential oils in the world are produced for flavorings or perfume, and they do not have a therapeutic effect. As use of oils becomes more popular, I believe we will see fewer false "certifications" and higher quality standards, due to more competition in the marketplace, and more organics will come to market.

I believe that essential oils are so popular because they've been marketed as an alternative to pharmaceuticals. (And America's honeymoon with the pharmaceutical industry is over. We've watched drugs claim lives of folks close to us and cure almost nothing. We're looking for something better.)

They're a quick, fairly inexpensive-per-drop way to aromatically or topically (or even internally, in some cases) raise our vibration.

Do your homework and know what is in your essential oils. Many claim to be "pure" when, in fact, independent labs show they have many synthetic chemicals in them. Those who sell them simply repeat the marketing information given to them by the manufacturer. Finally there are certified organic oils coming to market, and anything different than certified organic is nothing more than marketing claims.

Gary Young, founder of Young Living and widely considered the father of the modern essential oils movement, was measuring the vibrations of essential oils long before talk of vibration hit the mainstream. He measured basil oil at 52 Hz of energetic frequency, while other oils are even higher, including rose oil at an amazing 320 Hz. I am unaware of any other physical substance on earth with such a high frequency.

Organic essential oils, then, may be a part of your strategy to raise your ViQ. With high-vibe plants as your primary food sources, you may want to consider having on hand organic high-vibe plant oils as medicine as well.

The plant world holds the keys to many natural anti-inflammatory compounds, grounding compounds, and even cell-selective cytotoxic compounds that kill cancer cells but not healthy cells.

The world of plants provides many solutions that human beings and other living things can leverage to solve problems and to maintain health. After all, the father of modern medicine, Hippocrates, said, "Let food be thy medicine, and medicine thy food." We've strayed far from the idea that plants are our medicine, since the discovery that chemically altering a plant substance can make you a billion dollars.

(It is also true that synthetic drugs, virtually across the board, harm your vibration, as they are not natural substances and have very low frequencies. Your body does not assimilate or eliminate chemicals efficiently or completely, and residues build up in your organs and tissues and cause health issues.)

The essential oils industry is currently at $5 billion and is projected to be $12 billion by 2025. I do have a concern that, collectively, we're moving from a belief that a synthetic drug will solve our every problem to a slightly revised belief that a bottle of oil will solve our every problem.

Our base-level focus must be on an organic, mostly plant-based, whole-foods diet. Many among us, in the age of quick fixes, simply want something that requires no effort on our part.

So, while essential oils can be helpful, I hope you don't see them as the new "pill for every ill."

The 320 Hz rose oil is very expensive, of course, and makes a lovely perfume. But essential oils range from 50 Hz to more than 300 Hz, according to Young's research, and since oils are the highest-energetic part of the plant, it's a concentration in high vibration and may be a useful part of your goal to improve your grounding and your high, consistent, steady frequency.

::::: COFFEE, CAFFEINE, :::::
AND OTHER STIMULANTS

If a state of high vibration is still a bit of a unicorn for you and you aren't experiencing it on a regular basis, you may think of it as similar to the way you feel on stimulants.

High-vibration life is rather different—calmer, steadier, but energized. By contrast, a coffee or cola caffeine "high" is frenetic, and you may feel jittery, irritable, or anxious—plus there's the inevitable crash later.

Let's leave caffeine in highly unnatural soda and energy drinks in a separate category, where we acknowledge that it not only lowers vibration but also makes you sick, fills your cells with garbage, and damages your nervous system with neurotoxic chemicals that actually build up in the brain and cause headaches when you detox.

The soda and energy drinks absolutely have to go—worse than the caffeine are a dozen other toxic chemicals in those drinks.

Coffee, however, is considered a must by many cultures, and I don't believe I'll be successful at convincing many of my dear readers to give it up. So I'm going to attempt to put it in its place, weighing its positives and negatives, and then I'm going to give you some tips to mitigate the negatives of drinking it.

Coffee is hotly debated in the wellness space right now. With as many acidic compounds as coffee contains, as well as mycotoxins (molds) and loads of caffeine, not to mention the dairy products and refined sugar or chemical sweetener most people add, I disagree that its virtues outweigh its health hazards.

Of course, lots of positive press has come out about coffee in recent years, and that should be seen as what it is: marketing copy that shows up in the media because for-profit companies drive it there.

It's certainly true that I get more done on the occasions that I drink a cup of coffee. It also may be true that it dilates veins and ducts that cause you to eliminate more often and more completely.

However, when you rely on stimulants often, you are borrowing tomorrow's energy for today, and you have to continue the habit—which is, by definition, addiction.

The more free you are from addictions of every kind, the more in control of your own energies you are and the more capable you are of high-vibration living.

If you're going to drink coffee (and I don't think choosing decaf really makes a difference, as it's every bit as acidic and even more processed—and it still has some caffeine), here are nine tips to minimize the effects of your coffee-drinking habit:

1. Drink lots of water. Sometimes we are tired simply because we're dehydrated (which coffee/caffeine can cause, as it acts like a diuretic). Water will help to flush out the caffeine, rehydrate you, and restore the minerals that caffeine can deplete. If you require coffee or another stimulant source to be productive, consider increasing your water intake and see what happens. Or, at least, if you're going

to drink coffee, drink a cup of water with fulvic and humic acids in it as well.

2. Exercise can also help flush caffeine out of your body as well as help you burn off the jittery energy it causes. Aerobic activities such as swimming, biking, jogging, walking, Zumba, and hot yoga work best.

3. If you drink more than one or two cups of coffee a day, what if you decrease the quantity and replace it with much healthier green tea? Green tea is one of the highest-antioxidant beverages, full of catechins and other micronutrients—and it also contains natural caffeine. Some studies have suggested that catechins, which are antioxidant compounds, can help to reduce the risk of some diseases, such as cardiovascular and oral health problems, Alzheimer's, and certain cancers. Some also suggest they help promote weight loss, reduce body fat, and improve triglyceride levels.

4. If you accept the challenge I give you in this book of always having green juice or green smoothies on hand, consider drinking a glass of green juice before your coffee. This way, you are at least providing significant alkalinity to buffer the strong acids of your coffee.

5. Caffeine leaches vitamins out of the body, so eat your vitamins or take a good vitamin supplement. Because caffeine alters the whole-blood, plasma, and leukocyte levels that are regulated by vitamin C, it's especially important to get sufficient amounts of that vitamin through supplements or citrus foods.

6. Consider ditching the sugar and dairy or processed nondairy creamer. Instead, what about lightening your coffee with a tablespoon or two of full-fat coconut milk, which pro-

vides wonderful medium-chain triglycerides that are excellent for brain health, and adding a dropperful of liquid stevia or a spoonful of raw, organic coconut sugar? Other options are almond milk, cashew milk, and any other nut or seed milk. And other sweeteners include xylitol (still very processed but with little impact on blood sugar), raw honey, and coconut nectar.

7. Use organic, single-source-farmed coffee, which won't give you that jittery feeling and is sustainably and responsibly grown. Avoid Starbucks and the other coffee chains like the plague! Even their coconut milk is full of shoddy ingredients, their chai tea is just a sugary mix, their coffees are low-grade, and the syrup flavorings are really bad for you. These chains may be convenient, but they're not helping in upleveling your health and happiness through raising your frequency.

8. Eat a healthy meal to help your body absorb and break down the caffeine. Eating whole grains and leafy greens greatly helps this digestive process, as well as helping to put back the very important magnesium in your body that caffeine depletes.

9. Take a supplement that works to mitigate the negative effects of coffee/caffeine. L-theanine helps to normalize alpha brain waves, which become agitated when we are nervous, anxious, or jittery (common caffeine side effects), and also helps us relax, inducing a feeling of calm and general well-being.

:::: POLLUTION VERSUS OXYGEN :::: AND CLEAN AIR

More of us than ever live in cities, and it's a foregone conclusion that with millions of cars and lots of industry, the air we breathe isn't clean. I'm not going to take us through a depressing litany of all the chemicals we must breathe, both outdoors and indoors.

I myself live in what is, at least for a handful of days each year, one of the most polluted metropolitan areas in the world. The Utah and Salt Lake valleys experience a phenomenon called inversion, in which warm air traps cold air in the valley, usually during the winter. Until a strong wind and/or storm clears the air out, we are trapped in weeks of increasingly heavy pollution.

I buy a season pass to the Sundance Mountain Resort to ski, but that gets me out of the dirty air for only a few hours at a time, up Provo Canyon. And it leaves my children, in school or at work, down in the muck, which I worry about.

So this is one of the toughest ones, since it's hard to get away from and it's hard to mitigate. I like to plan my vacations to warm places or to clean places (like Hawaii or the Alps) for those winter months when inversion is likely.

My mother used to say, "I do all in my power, and then I pray to let grace take me the rest of the way." She said this with regard to how she lived through sending each of her eight children out into the world, some of them making poor choices and all of them encountering dangers every day. She put it in God's hands, but first she took precautions to teach us and armed us in every way possible.

Fear is very unhelpful to vibration, so while I do not like this one thing about the otherwise spectacular place where I live and have raised my four children, I embrace the realization that life has risk, and I choose to feel, think, and be in thoughts of health and empowerment and purity.

Every day, when you get a chance to be outside and when you go to yoga, practice taking thirty deep breaths. It will increase your lung capacity, after you've done this on a regular basis for a while. This gets oxygen to your bronchioles, those tiniest airways in the lungs—imagine them cleansing as you exhale and pinking up.

When I am feeling anxiety or fear, I take several deep breaths, reminding myself that "breath turns fear to excitement." It's been astonishing to me how this clears my anxiety and raises my vibe, and I can move forward with clean energy using such a simple technique.

Drinking lots of water, getting away to where the air is clean, and taking thirty deep breaths once a day will have a mitigating effect on the air pollution you are forced to breathe.

And know that I will pray for both you and me—and for our children—that this will be enough. Prayer, after all, is one of the greatest vibrational tools we have.

CHAPTER 6

Foods That Raise
(and Lower) Vibration

To give you a bit of inspiration and a suggestion of how broad the spectrum of ways you can shift your ViQ using food is, I've compiled a variety of data points in the bar chart below of the lowest- and highest-vibration foods, emotions, and substances, which can be measured in hertz. (Different scientists have measured vibration in other units, but because it is most familiar, I used data only from those measuring in hertz.)

The following data points were documented by the late Bruce Tainio, using his BT3 Frequency Monitoring System.

A healthy human being measures at 62 to 68 Hz. Remember that range, because it will be your reference point for what I'll explain next.

Extremely gifted, productive human beings have been measured at more than 80 Hz. Higher hertz are associated with health and happiness, and lower ones are associated with disease states, depression and anxiety, and low energy levels.

Tainio made these discoveries:

- Human cells mutate when their frequency drops below 62 Hz.
- Humans with a cold or the flu have 58 Hz of measured energy.

- A candida yeast overgrowth causes people to drop to 55 Hz.
- An Epstein-Barr virus patient has a frequency of 52 Hz.
- A cancer patient often has a frequency of 42 Hz or lower.
- The death process begins, for a human being, when frequency is measured at 25 Hz.
- Chicken and beef have only 2 Hz of energy. (They are, after all, dead flesh—and usually have been dead for a long time by the time you eat them.)
- Greens have 70 to 90 Hz of energy!

Remember what I said in the beginning of this book—the fourth principle you must understand as we discuss energetics and their impact on your life? *A substance with a higher frequency can cause the vibration of a substance with a lower frequency to increase.*

This is fabulously good news! Are you celebrating yet? Ready to put this into practice?

You should be, because what this means for you—no matter how tired, sick, and depressed you may be currently—is that you can change those lower states!

Literally just being in the presence of high-vibration people improves your own energetics.

Applying a high-vibration essential oil to the bottoms of your feet, to be instantly absorbed into the bloodstream, can raise your vibe. And drinking a green juice—whoa, look out, world!

As a public speaker, I can, with words and energy alone, completely transform the electricity in the room and uplevel virtually everyone there by many hertz. That's how powerful words, and word combinations, and positive thoughts, are. They are nothing more, and nothing less, than energies.

Now that you think of them that way, you can see how you can be a powerful agent for good or bad.

This bar chart by no means shows all the known measurements for frequencies of substances, emotions, and foods, but it gives you a graphic idea of how powerful the differences are between the bad guys and the good guys.

I hope you'll spend a few minutes with this chart and consider how much time and thought energy you put into fear and anger versus love and peace. When's the last time you had a pint of green juice versus a steak or chicken breast? When's the last time you used a drug to treat a symptom versus an essential oil or herb?

Just one more: When's the last time you did thirty minutes of yoga versus numbing out watching another dreadful, sarcastic sitcom or crime drama on TV?

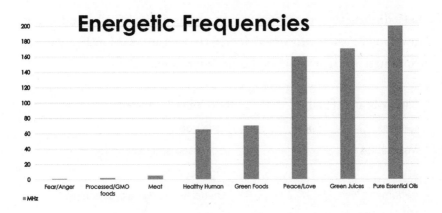

The amazing news here is that you don't need a complicated electrical frequency reader to know whether you're in a high-vibration state. You will know—because you'll simply feel amazing. You have intuitively sensed energies your whole life, whether you used those words for it or not.

When you discover the power of tuning in to and then tuning up your own and others' energies, you'll want to tell the world about it. (Now you know why I wrote this book!)

You'll want to document how and why your entire being feels electrically charged and, therefore, alive. You'll want to come back, again and again, to this place of optimal energetic frequency and make it your zone. It's your own Optimal ViQ.

I've written this book so that you'll learn how to be aware of your ViQ, how to achieve it, and how to protect it. For now, start to be aware of it—when it's low, when it's high, and why. You'll achieve lots of awareness about things you didn't understand before that are affecting your electrical frequency every day.

:::: PLANTS VERSUS ANIMALS, :::: LIVING VERSUS PROCESSED FOODS, AND OTHER COMPARISONS

Let's discuss the vibration of plant versus animal foods, and living, raw foods versus processed foods, as well as many other choices examined for their effect on human vibrational energy.

High-Vibration Foods	Low-Vibration Foods
Greens	Soda pop
Vegetables	Processed and canned foods
Fruits	Sugar and flour
Legumes	Animal flesh and dairy products
Whole grains	Coffee
Nuts and seeds	Chemical sweeteners (Splenda, NutraSweet, etc.)

In short, the most high-vibration diet features many plant foods, as shown in the pyramid ahead. While it does not show animal products, if you're going to eat them, make sure they're free-range, wild-caught, grass-fed, or organic. If I eat animal products, they are from clean sources that I know to have specific, well-documented health effects—such as organic, homemade kefir for its probiotics, or bone broth for its collagen and positive digestive-health effects. And I have a salad or green juice with almost every meal, for the enzymes and micronutrients that I need to balance out any animal proteins or less-than-ideal foods and keep my vibe high.

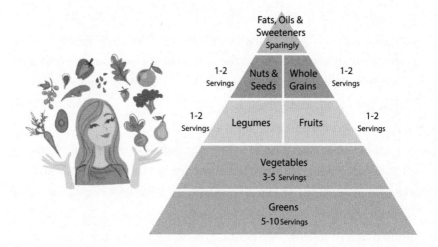

Many people trying to follow a program to get healthier accidentally end up in a low-vibration state because most diets are actually very low-frequency. A prime example of this is the processed whey protein shakes and bars that bodybuilders and fitness competitors eat lots of because they're really preoccupied with maxing protein and minimizing carbohydrates—which is a terribly low-frequency way to eat, causing rapid aging due to the lack of micronutrients in their excessive-protein diets.

You can tell if you look at their faces: check out YouTube videos of fitness competitors, especially men, who cannot cover it up with makeup. They routinely look ten years older than they are due to the typical bodybuilder diet.

Sure, they may have huge muscles, so in a way they're strong. But I've done muscle testing on guys who have a hundred pounds more muscle than I do, and they become total weaklings as you test the energy passing through their muscles when you put a cooked steak, or a cell phone, or a photo of their ex-wife in their hands!

The point is, you're not truly strong if you're not getting enough antioxidants to deal with all the free radicals that are the by-products of your musculoskeletal stress and the processed and dead-food diet you're on.

High-energetic ways to lose weight are far better than low-vibration ways. The standard American diet is the absolute worst, of course. But right behind it are the Atkins diet, the ketogenic diet that is trending right now (a variation on Atkins, but with a new preoccupation with fats), and—don't hate me for this—the Paleo diet. (That is, if you interpret paleo as "lots of meat.")

Studies show that people following the paleo diet are eating about 20 to 60 percent animal protein, compared to the average American, whose diet includes about 20 percent, or a healthy vegetarian who gets 10 percent protein. Some folks who claim to eat paleo are eating quinoa, beans, lots of veggies and greens, and less meat, but the vast majority are consuming excessive amounts of meat.

At least paleo lovers are avoiding dairy products and refined foods—we absolutely agree on that, the paleo advocates and I. But if we look at the very premise of this diet objectively, most of the humans in the Paleolithic era were eating the meat of mammoths, which are extinct, if they had access to meat at all, and lots of berries and greens and veggies that are no longer available thousands of years later. Many Paleolithic-era humans cultivated and ate grain in the fall and winter.

I'm a friend of doing the paleo diet if those following it tone down the meat eating, and some do. (Many humans in the Paleolithic era were actually eating a plant-based diet.)

A new food fad comes in every five to seven years, driven by the food industry. I wouldn't bet the farm on any of them. There's a better way to eat.

I don't push people toward a vegetarian or vegan diet, though that's what my own diet most closely resembles. I allow that my own daughter's 100 percent vegetarian diet may need some B_{12} and essential fatty acid supplementation, for instance, and perhaps something providing collagen, such as bone broth.

Millions of people eat a vegetarian diet the world over without supplementation (especially in Africa, India, China, Southeast Asia, and Central America). But in the modern world, many of us have deficits related to depleted soils or other issues with the microbiome (in the human gut) and toxins in our air and water that, inside us, cause metabolic problems.

Rather than adopt any -*isms*, I hope that if you do eat animal proteins, you eat only free-range, wild-caught, non-GMO eggs, and organic cuts of meat, and that you avoid dairy products (except ferments made from organic milk) like the plague that they are. And I hope that raw greens and lots of vegetables, some fruits, and some nuts, seeds, and legumes make up the bulk of what's on your plate.

I do believe that biodiversity is a fundamental consideration— we each have a different genetic makeup, and some may do well on a higher-protein diet while others do better on a vegetarian diet. Indeed, people all over the world thrive on both ends of the spectrum: folks who eat a significant amount of animal protein and vegetarians. Steering clear of dogmas and just looking at data leads us to this very evident conclusion: avoiding processed foods and eating a lot of plants seems to be the common thread in healthy diets where there is little associated disease.

All of us, regardless of our biological diversity, need to eat more greens. We need to eat more salads and more vegetables; more fibrous legumes such as split peas, lentils, and beans; and more gluten-free or low-gluten or non-hybridized grains or seed fruits (which resemble grains and cook like them), such as spelt, millet, amaranth, quinoa, bulgur, teff, and KAMUT.

:::: A NEW PARADIGM FOR :::: THINKING ABOUT FOOD

In this chapter, we will also discuss the ways we currently valuate food—and who taught us to think this way. (Hint: Big Food is a profit-driven industry, just like Big Pharma, and the dogmas you've been taught about food range from red herrings, at best, to outright harmful.)

I'll help you discover that the level of vibration that results from dietary choices and what you spend time thinking about can be far more powerful than the way you currently think. I'm talking about your thought patterns in your idle time—when you're driving, when you're in the shower, when you're walking the dog.

This is when you have your whole brain available to you, your idle time, and you can actually use it for massive upleveling. This is entirely different from being head-down on a project at work, where you're leveraging a specific part of your brain.

There are times during your day when you're using your whole brain—and, unfortunately, too many of us are using that time, mentally, to slowly destroy ourselves.

The level of vibration that results from various choices in your diet and everyday life may be the most relevant and helpful way to think of the consequences of those choices. After you've read this book, you should be forever changed in the way you look at all of the small, daily decisions you make, the way you spend your time, the ways you choose to medicate yourself, and the foods you select for your meals. You'll have a new construct and new language to evaluate those choices' impact on your quality of life.

However, industries have us thinking in "bunny trails," conditioned to believe in ways of measuring foods, choices, and dietary plans that do not serve us well—including you, probably.

More Useful and Sustainable than Calorie Counting

For instance, let's examine the concept of calorie counting. This is a valid but not particularly helpful way to analyze food choices. The idea is that high-caloric foods should be avoided if you're trying to lose weight, and high-caloric foods should be sought out if you're trying to gain weight.

This is problematic for a variety of reasons. First, calorie counting doesn't take into account the other useful properties a food may have, or the opposite—a complete absence of more important "food value."

Say you evaluate foods based on calories, with high calories being bad and low calories being good, as we have done for decades in the Weight Watchers program and many other—in fact, most—diet philosophies. In this construct, avocados are a bad food. In fact, avocados are one of the most perfect foods known to man.

If I had to choose three foods to have for the rest of my life on a deserted island, avocados would certainly be one of the them. Not only are they lovely to the taste, but they also have the most beneficial, fat-burning types of fats that the body needs for a healthy neurological system as well as a healthy heart to serve you well till you're a hundred.

If calories are the way you evaluate foods, you'll usually avoid fats altogether, since they have more calories per gram than carbs and protein.

We did, collectively, avoid fats altogether in the 1980s, to the detriment of our skin, our brains and nervous systems, and, really, the health, flexibility, and longevity of our every cell—each of which is protected by a lipid membrane made of the constituents of fats. People who avoid fats are aging more rapidly than necessary.

I deeply regret falling for that food cult when I was very young in the 1980s. Being duped by the food industry back then is part of why I'm on a mission to educate you against the guaranteed future shenanigans of the Big Food oligopoly. It teaches you whatever is in its marketing agenda, not the truth.

If you stay away from high-caloric foods, you'll avoid nuts, seeds, cold-pressed coconut oil, extra-virgin olive oil, and butter (one of the few dairy products that has health benefits)—and what a shame that would be. These are foods that have important virtues you can't get in the protein and carb worlds.

Let me give you another example of how the calorie obsession will steer you wrong, if that is your gold standard in evaluating choices at the grocery store.

Consider a bag of "low-calorie" chips: these may be mostly air, but they're also made of genetically modified corn, toxic refined salt, and diluted and highly refined oil. Everything about them lowers vibration and causes higher disease risk. It's a fake, processed, useless food. But it's low in calories, and many Americans, taught to evaluate foods based only on calories, consequently deem it a healthy one.

And if you read the package, they may have put some processed version of "protein" in the product, and the package may show what someone has told you is an optimal ratio of proteins, fats, and carbs. Never mind that there isn't a single natural ingredient in these chips.

Oh, and the serving size may be manipulated as well—as if anyone really eats six chips and puts the bag away! Keeping serving sizes unreasonably small can make you think, looking at the calories and the protein/fat/carb breakdown, that you're doing great.

So why are you still twenty pounds overweight, tired all the time, and foggy-brained every day?

I'd rather have you eat a higher-caloric, whole-food snack than a GMO, refined-salt, sugary corn-puff snack from a grocery store bag that says "low-calorie!" or "low-fat!"

Here's another example. I know a number of mothers whose very small children are suffering from being underweight. Sometimes they have severe asthma, as my son did, and are on many medications that affect their appetite. Others are diagnosed vaguely as "failure to thrive" and just aren't growing, and no one knows why.

In each case, doctors told the mothers to feed their children lots of ice cream and other fatty junk foods.

This reveals the ignorance of the medical profession about the consequences of our nutrition on our health beyond simply "calories in, calories out." Not all doctors and nurses, of course, are exclusively calorie- and macronutrient-obsessed, but those who do not educate themselves outside of what is taught in medical school often are. (A recent study shows that doctors' knowledge about nutrition is approximately the same as the knowledge of the average person on the street.)

For an asthmatic child, not much could be worse than feeding him dairy products full of sugar and hormones and the antibiotics fed to the cows. The fat molecule of the cow's milk is too big to cross the human semipermeable membrane easily, causing the body to produce mucus to flush it out. Therefore, dairy products like ice cream are a vibration-lowering, mucus-forming, poor food for the baby human, especially one struggling to achieve a normal weight.

The amount of fat in the food and its caloric density should not be the only factors we consider in feeding our children. What about micronutrients: enzymes, vitamins, minerals, and phytochemicals? What about fiber? What about vibrant colors (which are evidence of free-radical-neutralizing antioxidants), and how natural and unprocessed those foods are?

I don't think it will surprise you when I point out that the foods that are high in micronutrients and fiber, bright in color, and unprocessed are the foods that raise vibration too.

The processed-food industry has taught us to think in calories, grams, the ratios of the three macronutrients, and serving sizes. And not only is that system complicated, giving us a never-ending challenge (to count, measure, obsess)—it's not even serving us. We're fatter than ever, and we've got epidemics of heart disease, cancer, diabetes, and autoimmune disease—all lifestyle- and diet-related.

When we focus on the vibrational energy of the foods we choose, we literally build our cells out of higher-quality materials, so it follows that those cells can perform better. They vibrate at a higher speed and they are more impervious to cancer-causing agents.

And remember, *like attracts like.* So when you build your cells out of higher-quality materials, you are in turn attracted to higher-quality foods. You've heard of the downward spiral? This is the opposite of that: the upward spiral! You build your cells out of better materials, and they are then attracted energetically to better-quality materials (foods), and so on, until you are operating at a beautiful state of high vibration.

Then you aren't fighting constant internal struggles with wanting coffee, doughnuts, cigarettes, alcohol, soda, and chips. (I've just named possibly the six most low-vibration things many people consume.)

High-vibration folks simply aren't attracted to those things. If you are attracted to those things, don't feel bad—it's a journey, not a destination, and no one is perfect. Raising your vibration is a gradual process.

And I promise, if you just commit to the journey and to improvement, one day in the not-too-distant future, the things that tempt you daily right now . . . ? They won't be a problem. When you're several steps down the road from where you are now, they won't even appeal to you!

In my twenties, living my "low-vibration life," I ate a bag of York Peppermint Patties about every other day. (As a nod to that, I've posted a really funny video on your Resources page that I made with the "Ultra Spiritual" comedian JP Sears, in which he punches a bag of York Peppermint Patties out of my hand while teaching me to make a green smoothie with a yoga mat blended into it.)

For a while, I ate three frosting-covered chocolate doughnuts from a six-pack box every day. Corn syrup, chemicals, refined oils, sugar—everything about them was contributing to my low vibration. It was my daily treat, while my little kids took a nap.

I can't even remember the last time I ate a doughnut or a York Peppermint Pattie. Same thing goes for the pint of Ben and Jerry's ice cream my then-husband and I sat in a La-Z-Boy and ate, every night while I was pregnant, watching TV.

None of those things appeals to me now. This is something to celebrate, when foods that harmed your health and had power over you for many years don't anymore. That's one of the many triumphs of progressing toward higher and higher vibration.

In summary, I want to leave you with this important thought regarding the way you've been taught to evaluate food:

What if the energetic qualities, or vibrational energy, of the food we choose has far more to do with our health and well-being than calories, macronutrients, and serving sizes do?

More Useful and Sustainable than Macronutrient Obsession

Everyone in the Western world with a high school education knows that food is composed of fats, proteins, and carbohydrates. If that's all you know about food, academically, at least you know that.

This is the construct by which we understand food, and that's so because the mega-billion-dollar food industry wants us focused on this, as a red herring, so we don't easily come to the conclusion that the vast majority of what marketers are selling us is actually quite harmful.

That way, the big companies can simply manipulate macronutrients, change up the recommendations every decade or so, and reinvent everything. We, the poor consumers, then pore over packaging labels in the store, as we've been taught, to evaluate whether the "food" has enough protein and is low enough in carbs and calories. We stand there, feeling the anxiety about whether the fat grams are too high. Whether the ratios are right.

Those of us who lived through the 1980s may still have all kinds of discomfort about foods high in fat. (Never mind that some of the most perfectly proportioned human beings who have ever walked the planet are in the South Pacific, where, eating their native foods, their diet is about 65 percent fat! I'm not talking about the Pacific Islanders who live in Westernized cities; I'm talking about those in indigenous areas where the US is not importing much, if any, of their food—and what is imported, they can't afford or don't want. These people are not overweight.)

So, in the 1980s, the brilliant ploy of the food industry was to vilify fat. We then spent more than a billion dollars a year on low-fat and nonfat foods. Unfortunately, we would learn only after many years and billions of dollars out of our pockets that this was a terrible idea for our health. We would learn only through hard experience that our neurological health is harmed by lack of healthy, unprocessed fats in our diet. The kind found in nuts, seeds, very green extra-virgin olive oil, and even the much-maligned tropical oils, including the saturated-fat coconut oil!

We learned that everything we thought we knew about fat was wrong.

We have the Big Food oligopoly to thank for that. Did they reform? Are they now teaching us the truth, the whole truth, and nothing but the truth?

Unfortunately, no. They didn't, even after science caught up with them and ran the low-fat folks out of town. (Almost. Manufacturers still produce it, because some unfortunate people didn't get the memo and are still buying it.)

Those same huge companies simply reinvented themselves. What came next, as you know, was the low-carb craze.

For well over a decade, fats have been allowed back in the door and protein has been all but worshipped—but carbohydrates are now the villains.

We've been told we must avoid carbohydrates at all costs. Around the water coolers of America, many women have been heard to say things like this to their coworkers: "If I so much as look at a carb, it ends up on my thighs!"

Never mind the fact that most of our fuel since the dawn of time, for human beings—more than 60 percent, on average—has been carbohydrates. They are the preferred fuel of the liver.

And never mind the fact that when we throw out carbohydrates—the bad guys like white flour, white sugar, and concentrated sweeteners in general—we also throw out high-fiber, micronutrient-rich foods like sweet potatoes, oats, millet, carrots, beets, bananas, apples, and oranges.

These and many other wonderful high-carb foods give you energy and drag the digestive tract with lots of soluble and insoluble fiber to clean it and, consequently, your blood. They are well documented to be an important part of a disease-risk-minimized lifestyle.

And the recent trend, from Atkins to paleo, has been to vilify the mighty carbohydrate. That way, Big Food can launch a massive new trend worth billions annually all over again. Since the last cash cow died.

The next trend is already upon us, and I've been predicting it for a few years: the ketogenic diet, vaunting fat as the new "golden child" of macronutrients. It's an adjustment to Atkins, followed by paleo, that research is now saying doesn't really work and isn't particularly good for our health—not the way Americans are practicing it.

And as we've mentioned, the "paleo diet" has been debunked as having little or nothing to do with what Paleolithic man actually ate, if you accept that trying to copy what early hominids did is even a worthy goal. Many humans in the Paleolithic eras ate little animal meat, and none of them ate it two and three times a day, year-round, like those following the trendy diet usually do. And it's difficult or even impossible to eat meat, in the modern era, without steroids, hormones, and antibiotics, let alone the nitrates and nitrites curing agents. It's virtually impossible to avoid these, if animal products are a staple in your diet and if you ever travel or eat in restaurants.

Plus, most human beings in the Paleolithic age actually didn't eat meat but instead ate a high-grain, high-carb diet! The one thing that all Paleolithic humans had in common was that they didn't eat processed foods, and that's about all.

The ketogenic diet is starting to take over; it's actually just a new-old version of the thoroughly debunked Atkins diet, and it will be around for a number of years until science debunks it in turn—at which time another food cult will take over.

Taking a high-level view of nutrition history shows this pattern. Big Food is a mega-billion-dollar industry, and it absolutely must reinvent itself regularly to maximize profits. Carbohydrates will fall out of favor and make a comeback, and it's of little relevance if you want to eat healthy.

In fact, varying ratios of macronutrient percentages can lead to good health. Yes, that's right. You can eat more or fewer carbs, more or less protein, and more or less fat, and you don't have to live paralyzed by counting grams of various things. (You can't, anyway, with a lot of whole foods. Guess what—it's the packaged foods that have those measured for you, so no wonder the Big Food complex wants us obsessed with calories and protein/fat/carb grams and ratios! We then gravitate to their packages of more-or-less processed foods.)

How many grams of the three macronutrients, or calories, for that matter, does a banana have? Who knows! That depends on how big it is, how ripe it is, where it was grown, and who is measuring it. We haven't stamped bananas with all these fairly irrelevant pieces of data. (We can't. Bananas cannot be standardized—neither can anything else that grows in nature.)

What these labels do is keep us from paying attention to what actually matters.

How many grams of carbohydrates you eat is far less relevant than the type of carbs you eat!

For instance, a slice of Wonder Bread is a lousy carb, for sure. The manufacturer has used wheat that has likely been hybridized about two hundred times, making its gluten protein bizarrely inflammatory for the human body, even if it makes a fluffy, soft bread.

And they're not done yet making it truly junk. They then strip out all the vitamins and minerals found in the germ of the wheat. And they throw away the bran, where all the fiber is.

Now it's a nutritionally empty "Frankenfood" that's likely to leave you bloated, with gluey gunk in your intestines slowing your digestion and your overall energies.

But steel-cut oats are carbs too; your oatmeal is full of fiber and micronutrients and are a healthy food, as shown in many studies. If all you do is look at labels, you'll get little or no sense of that, and we've been trained by the Big Food complex to evaluate food in this way.

My point is that how many calories—or what percentage or how many grams of carbohydrates you eat today—is a bunny trail, and the real story is told in the quality or the source of your carbs.

Fruits and vegetables are full of carbs. And they're the antidote to the standard American diet and all the destruction and havoc that have resulted from it.

Eating fruit has not been linked to diabetes risk. But only when you strip all the fiber and other nutrition out of that piece of fruit and drink it in concentrated form or add quantities of refined sugar in its many forms to your food does it become, over time, an insulin problem that compromises your health.

(This is not to say that those with diabetes don't need to count their carbs. After you've been diagnosed, that may be necessary. But my point here is that we could all avoid the ongoing type 2 diabetes epidemic—which some experts say will have as much as one third of us diagnosed within the next thirty years—if we eat the whole fruit instead, not the fruit juice and all the other sugary, altered, unnatural variations.)

What about fats? Are they the devil? You'd think so, if you were around in the 1980s like I was. We were told to avoid saturated fats at all cost, and tropical oils like coconut oil and palm oil were driven out of the food supply.

Our resulting deficit in medium-chain fatty acids may have played a role in the subsequent meteoric rise in neurological diseases such as multiple sclerosis, Parkinson's disease, ALS (Lou Gehrig's disease), Alzheimer's, and dementia. Because, it turns out, those dreaded whole-food saturated fats are important for brain and nervous system health, and Pacific Island cultures that eat a native diet containing them have very low rates of disease.

Other fats like extra-virgin olive oil, rich in polyphenols and essential fatty acids like omega 3s, are absolutely critical for cardiovascular as well as neurological health, and there's evidence that good fats help burn bad fats!

But, of course, frying potatoes in refined vegetable oil is a completely different thing: it's toxic, it clogs your arteries, it has no redeeming value, and it actually causes a lot of free-radical damage and inflammation in our cells.

That's a far cry from what the Big Food machine taught us in the 1980s—that fats are to be avoided! That their refined, often GMO "vegetable" oil is good for you.

So, again, how many grams of fat you eat or how many calories come from fat matters little compared to the quality of the fat.

As for protein, there's a huge qualitative difference between the protein of a Frankenfood egg, or a hot dog, or farmed fish versus a wild-caught salmon from clean waters.

That conventional egg has far too much omega 6 and far too little omega 3, leading to an imbalance for most Americans and putting us at high risk for heart disease.

The hot dog is full of all manner of animal parts you don't want to think about—but even worse are the nitrites and nitrates, which are the most carcinogenic food additives out of about five thousand the FDA has approved.

Farmed fish are dangerously loaded with heavy metals, which do neurological damage and cause autoimmune disease.

So, again, the quantity of the macronutrient—whether protein, fat, or carb—is less relevant than the quality.

High-quality materials build high-vibing cells, tissues, and organs!

An End to Dieting and Confusion

The world of fake processed foods, with its complicated valuation and measurement strategies, wants you confused.

Many industries want your focus on grams and calories.

The conglomerate of powerful food industries that supply most of what Americans eat also wants to control the way you view your food, the very system that tells you how to make choices.

Think about it. The cereal industry makes $1 billion or more a year. Ditto the dairy industry. The refined-flour industry. The sugar cane industry. The canned-food industry. The fast food industry—think of all the suppliers of products, equipment, buildings. It's big money. These companies are heavily leveraged, with warehouses, equipment, elaborate distribution channels, tall buildings full of employees making the whole machine go. Boards of directors and shareholders to answer to.

And with big money comes big marketing spending. Most of the "information" you encounter on the Internet and elsewhere was manufactured for you by these industries—just like they manufacture the food you eat. Most "information" now is really just marketing.

They pay researchers to do "studies" where only favorable information comes to light; they pay writers and public relations professionals and ad agencies; and they buy advertising on Facebook, TV, and in many other places.

But when you emerge into the light and out of the confusion, with the clarity that high-value food came to life under the sun, with its roots in the soil and clean water nourishing it, and without exposure to chemicals—you'll never be the same. You'll actually begin to free yourself from the brain damage that results from trying to learn how to eat from the media.

You won't need to go on diets. Or count anything. You'll be able to trust your body and your appetite and eat as much as you want. Because what you want will have changed.

And when you eat or drink something green, you're thinking about the chlorophyll, which is about to land in your body as a veritable blood transfusion, mopping up free radicals. And you are energetically attracted to it with your new awareness. And because you're made of higher-vibration materials, you're attracted to higher-vibration foods.

It's a process, increasing your vibration. It's built on discoveries and experimentation. I'm not going to ask you to take my word for it—that rebuilding your body, cell by cell, will literally change your tastes for food, will make you want more of the good and less of the bad, will have you ecstatic instead of depressed.

I'm simply going to show you a seven-day process wherein you will discover it for yourself.

You'll see how your body reacts when it is supplied only high-vibration food. It may not mean you never make a low-vibration choice again, since most of us learn in a "two steps forward, one step back" manner.

But this seven-day process will absolutely turn on lots of light-bulbs for you about what kinds of foods raise your mental clarity, creativity, energy, productivity, and enthusiasm. All for the possibility that when you bathe every cell in high-vibration foods only, your love and respect for all life increases, as well as your ambition. Making these connections can't help but improve your choices.

As Oprah says, "When you know better, you do better."

Yes, food has everything to do with all of those things. And we'll prove it, with our very own personal science experiment, where you are the test subject!

It's a bonus that you'll likely ditch five pounds, your bad mood, and your achy joints—all in just seven days. Are you ready?

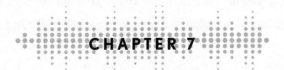

CHAPTER 7

The 7-Day High-Vibration Detox

Are you ready to lose five pounds this week and ditch your bad mood and achy joints?

In 2013, after almost three years of work, I launched the Green-SmoothieGirl detox program. I had researched, for twenty years, the detoxification systems of the body and the work of great doctors and researchers who have discovered how to purify the human tabernacle, which becomes increasingly important the dirtier the environment we live in becomes. The average baby is now born with well over two hundred synthetic chemicals, many of them known toxins, in the umbilical cord. And that's just from gestation, before she even draws her first polluted breath.

The fact is, many Americans have never skipped a meal. They virtually never experience hunger. The statement "I'm starving" is tossed around when the lunch hour nears at work and colleagues are discussing which restaurant to hit today. But the Western world, which is likely where you are reading this book, currently published only in English, knows nothing of hunger.

It's not that you have to be hungry to do the detox. You don't, whether you're doing the full, longer program or the shorter, seven-day experiment that I'm challenging you to undertake here!

But when you're opting out of your comfort foods, your stimulants, your daily sugary treat, and your drive-thru, it can initially feel like deprivation.

So, we're going to set some intentions toward having a fantastic learning opportunity, as well as a very effective house-cleaning. Let's set intentions toward letting go of what is not serving you and is currently cluttering up your critical organs' ability to do a perfect job for you every day.

:::: DETOXER OBSERVATIONS I DIDN'T EXPECT ::::

But first I want to share some amazing discoveries I uncovered, now that more than ten thousand people have completed our detox programs (the longer version and this short version I share with you here).

In the previous chapter, I explained what foods are featured in the detox program and why. That is, we eat almost entirely greens, vegetables, fruits, nuts, seeds, legumes, and non-hybridized whole grains.

I also explained what low-vibration foods are—and of course they are eliminated in your seven-day cleanse. These are animal proteins, coffee, soda, sugar, flour, alcohol, salt, and all processed food.

When I designed the detox, I was highly focused on physical benefits. You can see, at a glance, that the foods that raise vibration are high in fiber. They are natural, and you can buy and prepare them or eat them plain. They aren't processed, with the nutritious parts removed, and offered only in a box, bag, or can. Many, if not most, are found in the produce section of the grocery store. They are high in micronutrients: enzymes, vitamins, minerals, and phytochemicals.

So you would expect that eating only these foods for a period of time would involve digestive changes—usually larger stool eliminations and perhaps softer or even looser stool. You would expect that without sugar and gluey, high-gluten grain products, meat and dairy products, and stimulants, sustainable energy would increase. (This is different from bouncing-off-the-walls, coffee-induced "energy.")

You might anticipate that people would lose weight. And that inflammation would decrease for many and their joints would feel better.

All of these hypotheses proved to be true. We have had data pouring in for more than four years now from hundreds of respondents who completed the detox programs. I read every single questionnaire, so let me share the results. Because you'll be doing a seven-day slice of that program, so you can expect some of these results yourself.

For instance, in the full 26-Day Detox program, the average participant loses more than twelve pounds! And participants can eat as much as they want of a number of foods. The average detoxer finds more mental clarity, inflammation disappears, and formerly aching joints feel great. Energy increases for most.

But what was astonishing to me and my team, in evaluating the results that came in, was the additional comments detoxers shared with us about other areas of their lives that improved with this nutrition-focused change in their lives. Things outside the realm of the physical.

One-on-one, when I was just out in public or when I was in hundreds of cities on my lecture tour, people shared miracles far beyond pounds lost or brain fog cleared.

They spoke of their sex lives improving, with a causal effect in improving their marriages. Increased energy translated into more motivation to give more in family and other relationships.

They told me stories of their teenage children's grades improving during the teens' participation in the program, because they were able to focus.

Participants reported a significant change in their attitudes—toward the detox itself later in the process, toward their life and their work, toward the people they live and work with.

Detoxers have also reported to me, in person and in our written questionnaires, feeling more productive, positive, and even ambitious than they had in years, sometimes decades, and getting long-neglected projects done.

In 2009, I also did some research with 175 people who started a green smoothie habit. Green smoothies are not all you eat, but they feature prominently in this 7-Day Detox. Not because they're the only way to get greens into your diet, but because they're the easiest way to get in many servings of the greenest, most nutritious foods available to you. (In just one quart, you're going to get about ten servings of plants!) So this is relevant to you, as I hope a quart a day of "very green" smoothie is a lifelong practice that the detox inspires you to do!

To be a part of my 2009 study, people had to be drinking at least a pint a day of green smoothie at least four days a week. Many who participated were drinking more than that. For virtually everyone, it was a new habit, as they were following the new GreenSmoothieGirl .com site I had put up in 2007 when there were only fifty searches a month, worldwide, for the term "green smoothie." (Now it is almost a household term, and since my book released, at least a hundred other folks have jumped on the bandwagon and published green smoothie books.)

I often drink two quarts a day of green smoothies, or green juice delivered by a juice shop nearby—part of my ongoing assist for my body's daily detoxification processes. In fact, I even take frozen pints of green juice on trips, because they keep well that way, and I can stretch them to last three days away from home as they thaw—and in addition to packing some in luggage, I can even take a frozen pint through airport security. (After all, it's not a liquid!)

If that seems like too much for you, that's okay. Right now, we're just aiming for a dedicated seven days. After that, check out your

Resources page for ideas on how to keep your engine running clean, with minimal time in the kitchen, for life!

The results of the study were very exciting, and I submit them to you as evidence of high-vibration results when you eat high-vibration foods in much higher quantities than you do now.

Research Statistics

The following are some of the statistics that come from my research.

Reported Health Benefit	% of Participants
More energy	85%
Better digestion	79.5%
Fewer cravings for sweets/processed foods	65%
Skin clearer, improved skin tone	50%
Weight loss (some participants did not need weight loss)	50%
More positive/stable mood	54%
Higher libido	20%
Increased desire for exercise	46%
Improved sleep (need less, less insomnia, more alert in morning)	45%
Feel less stressed-out	44%
Stronger fingernails	37%
Shinier hair/no dandruff	27.5%
Blood sugar stabilized	39%
Decreased PMS symptoms (not all respondents were premenopausal women)	22%

In our extensive testing, we have been astonished and gratified to see that by increasing intake of high-vibe foods and eliminating the processed ones, plus putting some practices in place throughout the program, detoxers achieved high-frequency results often far beyond their wildest dreams. This program leverages the greatest known principles of human detoxification that virtually anyone can do.

:::: HEALTH BENEFITS OF DETOXING ::::

In addition to the emotional release that often accompanies detoxing, let me share a few things that may get you excited about undertaking this experiment!

Extra water, and hence less work for the liver, means you can release bile and flush it out—clearing toxins trapped in the liver. Since the liver has at least five hundred functions, letting it clean house is obviously a positive thing that can benefit you in hundreds of ways!

The kidneys may be cleansed of acids and even crystals that could potentially cause you problems with kidney stones later, and it is a logical inference that such a cleanse now and then makes outcomes like that far less likely.

The blood naturally becomes cleaner when the gastrointestinal tract is clean, with active, pink tissues and active peristaltic action, clearing the heavy mucoid plaque clogging it. That's because the blood circulates throughout the entire body every four minutes. So, when there's old junk in the colon, it circulates and recirculates those toxins in the bloodstream, and the liver does the best it can to filter. All toxic by-products of food and chemical exposure that leave the body allow the colon, blood, liver, and kidneys to run cleaner!

The lymphatic system too—the counterpart to the bloodstream, which "takes the trash out" after the blood "brought the groceries in"—can become more active when it is cleansed of debris. At first, of course, as there is increased throughput, some systems can become temporarily backed up. That's why in the detox itself, we give you tips to get things moving, to facilitate throughput.

Each individual has a unique, specific reaction to the program, either the seven-day version in this book or the more detailed full detox on GreenSmoothieGirl.com. For some, the reactions can be as much an emotional catharsis as a physical cleansing of the body.

The work of Dr. Richard Anderson taught me many years ago that emotions, even those far in your past, are trapped in physical proteins in tissues and cells. As you cleanse the various organs of your body, matter that may have been trapped there even for years, such as mucoid plaque in the colon and intestines, evacuates the body, and occasionally the person feels those emotions all over again as it departs.

I thought this was a very strange concept when I read it many years ago. I had not yet learned that all matter is in motion, that all physical "things" are nothing more nor less than energies. I wasn't sure I believed that, since it sounded undocumented and very new-agey.

So now that I understand more fully, it makes perfect sense, the idea of "feelings" being energies trapped in proteins. Hopefully, by this point in this book, it makes sense to you as well!

I experienced the truth of this once myself, during a very dedicated cleanse I did for a few weeks. In one particular experience during those days of eliminating the buildup or consequences of my standard American diet, as matter was leaving my body, I felt a sudden and overwhelming flood of old feelings about a family member who had physically and emotionally abused me as I was growing up.

I felt the fear, the anger, the grief, and a rush of memories of how this person had wronged me, a tidal wave of emotion that very nearly swamped me. Except that, after a minute or two, that rush of emotion and memory left me. It left me completely. I was able to write this family member a letter, forgiving her completely, and the feelings of anger and resentment never returned. This, all by itself, was worth doing that program—because I'd struggled with feelings about it (and her) my entire life.

When it was complete, I was a believer. I was fascinated by what had just happened, which was far deeper than the physical effect, and I was highly motivated to never again have clearly years-old, toxic material like that anywhere in my body. I wanted to make sure my body ran cleaner in the first place, and I wanted to make sure that I did periodic dedicated cleanses.

I studied extensively for many years. I learned about how many chemical agents—with properties that are carcinogenic, radioactive, and causative for autoimmune disease—are in the average human body.

I began to learn how many of them came from common food additives approved by the FDA. Our chemical exposure comes in common cosmetic and personal-care products and fragrances, in carpeting, inside cars, in industrial pollution, in additives like chlorine and fluoride in municipal water, in plastics that our food and water arrive in, in residue of the pharmaceutical drugs we've taken, in electromagnetic frequencies from our devices.

It could be rather depressing, except that I was also learning how to avoid most of the exposure, and to give my body a chance to eliminate much of the toxicity.

It became extremely clear that detoxing was as nonnegotiable for my health as it is for a cocaine or heroin addict. I don't smoke crack, but I accidentally ingest hundreds of other chemicals in any given year. Through air, water, food, and even the by-products of metabolism of even healthy food that my body is performing every day.

The most straightforward health benefit of making digestion very easy for your body is that a clogged colon and intestinal tract can release old materials. Many of us have hardened material, which Dr. Bernard Jensen called "catarrhal mucoid plaque," in the thirty to thirty-five feet of our gastrointestinal tract.

People who eat a typical American diet featuring things like white-flour products and significant amounts of animal proteins, which have no fiber and can be glue-like in the long human GI tract, are highly prone to this buildup of plaque.

People often say they eliminate every day, so they aren't constipated. But it's not what's coming out that's the problem—it's what's *not* coming out! People should ideally eliminate three times a day, after each meal.

When we devote time to the liver in the longer detox, we assist it in releasing toxins and flushing bile, clearing residue often trapped in the liver. You will get an abbreviated version of this in the 7-Day Detox in this book.

In the longer program, acids and even crystals that could cause problems later are eliminated safely and without pain. "Cleaning house" occasionally makes outcomes like kidney stones far less likely. We need a more extended period of time to get to this phase: for you, while reading this book, we want you to experiment for a short time with what cleansing is like, and what its benefits for you may be.

Detox Reactions

A majority of detoxers describe some kind of Herxheimer reaction, which is a classic response when output dramatically increases, in the blood, lymph, colon, and other pathways, and causes discomfort or blockages—a brief "retoxing"—on its way out.

The most common detox symptoms are, first, headaches, especially if you're a caffeine drinker (soda, energy drinks, or coffee).

Next is low energy. While increased energy is a long-term effect of detoxing, some people do experience lower energy for a short time—and even, for a few, all the way through the process.

If this happens to you, it's generally because you have more difficult health issues and higher levels of toxicity. When heavy metals and highly toxic chemicals, such as those used in chemotherapy, begin to come out of the body, sometimes you experience a very mild form of what you did when it went in!

I often say, using a chemo drug as an example, "Methotrexate goes in hard, and comes out hard!" (Former chemo patients who detox often describe a metallic taste in their mouths, even if the treatment was many years previous—proof positive that bad stuff comes out when the right good stuff comes in, as well as proof that the body does harbor heavy metals and other chemicals that need assistance to be eliminated.)

Third, digestive changes can be a result: diarrhea, increased frequency, or occasionally the opposite of that, temporary constipation. Anytime you radically change your diet, the body has a response time, and speeding up or slowing down elimination can be a temporary result!

Also, a small number of detoxers may find they have swollen lymph nodes, or their skin breaks out, or their teeth feel fuzzy. These are typical Herxheimer reactions as more gunk is leaving the body and you can see or feel the effects in skin, colon, lymph, or other systems.

Still, it's an important process to eliminate these terribly destructive chemicals that are harbored in organs and tissues and continue their damage.

It's a good process, despite a bit of discomfort for some; so be aware, tap into the tips above to clear blockages more quickly, and accept that your body is doing what it needs to. Drink extra water, rest more if needed, and be patient with the process, if you experience any "cleansing crisis" or detox reactions.

:::: WHY AM I EATING THESE :::: PARTICULAR FOODS?

The meals I have chosen and the recipes I have developed are very purposeful. The menus and recipes are intended to be easy, with few ingredients, and high-intolerance foods have been eliminated. Every single ingredient is easy for the body to digest, alkalizing, oxygenating, high in fiber, and nutrient-dense.

As billions of cells eliminate toxins and begin operating at optimal frequencies, you will feel it. You will know something energetically magical is happening, in the collection of vibrations that has organized, uniquely, as YOU!

You will accomplish a wonderful start toward optimizing your ViQ, partly because you will be eating high-fiber foods. Insoluble fiber drags the colon like a broom or scrubber, and gel-like soluble fiber lets you absorb and remove toxins. And you are flooding the body with vitamins, minerals, phytonutrients, and enzymes that your cells mop up and use to rid the body of free radicals.

Calories will be lower than your normal intake, to let the digestive system rest from its normal dedication to metabolism. This allows energy to be redirected to cleansing and repair work. You can eat as much as you want of many of the things in the program, and you don't need to worry about overeating. When you're satisfied or even full, you're full of fiber and low-calorie, nutritious food that absolutely won't cause you to gain weight.

CHAPTER 8

The 7-Day Detox Plan

This chapter lays out very specific meal plans, with a way to avoid ever getting hungry, so that anyone can succeed. The meals I have chosen and the recipes I have developed are very purposeful. Every single ingredient is easy for the body to digest, alkalizing, high in fiber, and nutrient-dense. The menus and recipes are intended to be easy, with few ingredients, and the recipes do not contain ingredients that are common allergens. No table salt of any kind is allowed, in order to flush excess sodium (which causes water retention and inflammation) from the cells. Some of the foods are purposefully rich in potassium, increasing the potassium-to-sodium ratio.

(Don't worry, there is natural sodium, the element that you need, in your food—table salt, or NaCl, is toxic, and doing without it for seven days helps you "reset.")

You're eating no animal flesh and no dairy products, except for some salt-free, organic butter—and the rest of the program is organic plant foods. Everything you'll eat for seven days is high in both soluble and insoluble fiber, alkaline-forming in the body, oxygenating, highly cleansing, and nourishing. You're eating no processed food, no toxic or refined sugars, no coffee or caffeine, and no neurotoxins or other chemicals, such as aspartame or monosodium glutamate (MSG).

We aren't trying to make you a vegan, just because you're eating plant foods for a week. If you do return to your meat-eating diet after this short reboot, it's extremely important not to eat processed meats like hot dogs, lunchmeats, bacon, sausage, and pepperoni.

And most meat products you will purchase, even if they don't have nitrites and nitrates in them—which are highly toxic and carcinogenic and found in processed meats—still have antibiotics, steroids, hormones, and GMO corn by-products that the animal ate.

Similarly, if you resume eating animal products after the detox, please avoid most dairy products, including cheese, milk, and ice cream, which are highly inflammatory and mucus-forming in the body—and also avoid pork, which is very dirty and prone to parasites and larvae.

Eat only organic, free-range eggs, and wild-caught or organic poultry, fish, steak, and bison, as they are your cleanest sources of animal protein. And make them a minor part of your meal, with the biggest part being whole plant foods such as salads, raw or cooked veggies, nuts and seeds, and legumes like lentils, split peas, and beans.

::::: DAILY PRACTICES TO ENHANCE ::::: YOUR DETOX

In addition to the diet, there are several principles and habits I'd like to review with you before you get started. They are important to understand so that you can commit to them. It's important to do several things (or as many as you can) noted in the list below *every day* during the detox, plus two that are optional but very helpful. And there are also three things to studiously *not* do.

Make Sure You DO:

- Skin-brush. (See your Resources page for a video demo.)
- Drink nine glasses of water.
- Massage your colon, with a tennis ball or your hands, morning and night.
- (Optional) If at all possible, spend thirty minutes in an infrared sauna.
- (Optional) If at all possible, take a home enema or professional colonic at any time, especially toward the end of the seven days. One per day, during the last one to three days, should be enough.

Make Sure You DO NOT:

- Eat more than 10 mg/serving of salt (inherently found in any packaged food).
- Eat any food after 7 p.m. (this gives the body a twelve-hour break from digestion, an important part of the detox).
- Eat the following:
  - Alcohol, caffeine, tobacco, stimulants, coffee or tea with caffeine
  - Dairy products including milk, cheese, yogurt, etc. (organic unsalted butter is allowed)
  - Eggs
  - Sugars and sweeteners (including sugar, fructose, Sucanat, coconut sugar, sucralose, xylitol, cane juice, rice syrup, agave, corn syrup, honey, molasses, date sugar, maple sugar)
  - White flour, white rice, white pasta
  - Yeast
  - Animal flesh: pork, beef, bison, elk, venison, lamb, veal, turkey, chicken, goose, duck, fish, shellfish, crus-

taceans, mollusks, any processed meats (which are the worst, including hot dogs, sausage, bacon, luncheon meats, corned beef, pastrami, salami, and ham)

* Monosodium glutamate (MSG), NutraSweet (aspartame), and all food additives and chemicals
* Mushrooms
* Pepper (a gastrointestinal irritant)

:::: YOUR DETOXIFYING DAILY ROUTINE ::::

As part of your daily routine, do the following:

• Before you get out of bed, massage the transverse colon for a few minutes.

Ideally you will have a tennis ball next to your bed to massage your abdomen deeply, but if not, use your fingers to press into your lower right abdomen, inside the pelvic bone. In a circular motion, massage straight up, and then over to the left under the navel, and straight down on the left side next to the pelvic bone, then back to the right; repeat.

This "wakes up" the peristaltic activity and contributes to healthy muscle tone and function in the large intestine. If you encounter a tender area, this may be an area of blockage you should spend a little extra time massaging.

• Drink about 1 ounce of water for every 2 pounds of weight.

So if you weigh 150 pounds, drink about 75 ounces of water each day. That's nine glasses!

• To help your lymph system "take out the trash," do either or both of the following:

- Spend 5 minutes skin-brushing, to increase lymph circulation and clean skin pores to improve detoxification through multiple avenues. (For a visual demonstration, see your Resources page for a video showing exactly how to skin-brush.)
- Jump for at least five minutes on a rebounder. Massage your lymph system in short, light strokes as you jump. On the sides of your neck, massage upward using your fingers. Massage the sides of your torso, from low to high. Rub the sides of your breasts, from bottom to top, on the outside, in brisk strokes.

- Spend thirty minutes in an infrared sauna, if possible.

Start at a temperature of 130°F to 140°F if you have not built up a tolerance. A temperature of 150°F to170°F is beneficial after you have used the sauna several times.

See the Resources page for a video of me showing my own infrared sauna and why I consider it an important tool in my detoxification arsenal.

::::: SUGGESTIONS FOR SUCCESS :::::

- Line up a buddy! Consider having someone else geographically close to you join you, as an accountability partner and for sharing food prep. Support each other in any challenges and successes.
- Shop one or two days before you intend to begin the detox.
- Plan for two hours of preparing food the day before you begin the detox. This will make those first four days very easy. When all the food requiring more than five minutes of prep time is made in advance, you will not find your-

self ravenously hungry with twenty minutes or sixty minutes of cooking to do. (That's deadly to your willpower!) Having the food available as you begin to feel hunger is the key to staying with it.

- You may feel absolutely stuffed trying to eat the portions prescribed, especially breakfast and lunch. Trust me, as counterintuitive as this sounds, just do it! The meals are so low-calorie, you may still be hungry by the next meal.

- Should you feel hungry late at night (your all-vegetable dinner will digest before bedtime), use only the legal cheats—for instance, a scoop of organic, plant-based protein powder in water, or a large spoonful of chia seeds stirred into a tall glass of water (drink it quickly). In ten to fifteen minutes, your hunger pains will be gone! That's because not only is chia low in calories and high in many nutrients, including protein and iron and vitamin C, it also absorbs ten times its own weight in water, so it becomes filling as it absorbs the water in your stomach. It's a habit you might find yourself retaining after the detox!

- Eat your next meal or snack when you first begin to feel hungry. Don't wait until you are extremely hungry—that is a sure way to feel discouraged and deprived.

- You can add up to two scoops of raw, vegan, organic plant-based protein to each quart of green smoothie. Plus you can have extra "protein shakes" of a scoop mixed in water at any time of day.

:::: MENU PLAN: DAYS 1 TO 4 ::::

Breakfast

- 1 quart Classic Green Smoothie (with optional 2 scoops raw, organic, plant-based protein and optional 1 scoop of sprouted flax, for essential fatty acids)

Lunch

- 1 quart Classic Green Smoothie (with optional 2 scoops raw, organic, plant-based protein and optional 1 scoop of sprouted flax)

NOTE: You can switch the foods eaten at lunch and dinner, if you'd like.

Dinner

- Days 1, 3: Lentil Soup and Cucumber-Tomato Salad
- Days 2, 4: Baked potato (with 1 to 2 tablespoons organic, unsalted butter) and Purple Heaven

Legal Cheats!

Snacks to ward off hunger anytime:

- Lemonade made with water, fresh lemon juice, and stevia to taste
- Water with 1 tablespoon chia seeds stirred in, up to three times a day (very filling!)—or put the chia in the lemonade above
- Protein shake made with 1 scoop raw, vegan, organic protein (nothing else added, except chia is legal)

:::: MENU PLAN: DAYS 5 TO 7 ::::

Breakfast

- Days 5 and 6: 1 quart Hot Pink Breakfast Smoothie
- Day 7: Breakfast Oatmeal and 1 pint Classic Green Smoothie (with optional 1 scoop raw, organic, plant-based protein and optional ½ scoop of sprouted flax)

Lunch

- Days 5 and 6: Baked sweet potato (with 1 to 2 tablespoons organic coconut oil) and 1 pint Classic Green Smoothie (with optional 1 scoop raw, organic, plant-based protein and optional ½ scoop of sprouted flax)
- Day 7: Black and Green Salad and 1 pint Classic Green Smoothie (with optional 1 scoop raw, organic, plant-based protein and optional ½ scoop of sprouted flax)

Dinner

- Days 5 and 6: Crunchy Avocado Salad and 1 pint Classic Green Smoothie (with optional 1 scoop raw, organic, plant-based protein and optional ½ scoop of sprouted flax)
- Day 7: Black and Green Salad and 1 pint Classic Green Smoothie (with optional 1 scoop raw, organic, plant-based protein and optional ½ scoop of sprouted flax)

Legal Cheats!

Same as before!

::::: SHOPPING LIST :::::

NOTE: Bunch units are based on medium-size bunches, but sizes vary widely, so keep an eye on what you are buying. But if you happen to have leftover greens, remember that they can be washed and then frozen in plastic freezer bags to be used in green smoothies later.

Food Item	Notes & Tips	Unit	# of People on Detox			
			1	2	3	4
Produce						
organic greens	choose from spinach, chard, kale, collards, beet greens, cabbages, etc.	bunch (see note above)	8	16	24	32
apples	organic if possible		4	8	12	16
bananas			6	12	18	24
medium beets			2	4	6	8
large avocado	organic if possible		2	4	6	8
celery		stalk	5	12	17	22
baking potatoes			2	4	6	8
sweet potatoes			2	4	6	8
small red onions			1	1	1	1
large yellow onions			3	6	9	12
green onions		bunch	2	4	6	8
green cabbage		small head	1	2	3	4
purple cabbage		small head	1	2	3	4
organic large carrot			5	10	15	20
medium lemons	for Avocado Salad, add more for legal cheat		1	2	3	4
limes	¼ cup juice needed per person; freeze any extra		3	6	9	12
garlic		clove	3	6	9	12
organic cucumbers			2	4	6	8

Food Item	Notes & Tips	Unit	# of People on Detox			
			1	2	3	4
organic medium ripe tomatoes			4	8	12	16
organic ripe Roma tomatoes	or 2/3/4/5 large regular		3	6	9	12
fresh cilantro		bunch	2	3	4	5

Canned Goods

Food Item	Notes & Tips	Unit	1	2	3	4
tomato sauce	low-salt or no-salt-added	small can	1	2	3	4
coconut water/juice	NOT coconut milk	12-ounce can	2	4	6	8
black beans		12-ounce can	1	2	3	4

Frozen Items

Food Item	Notes & Tips	Unit	1	2	3	4
strawberries	organic if possible	12-ounce bag	2	4	6	8
mixed berries	organic if possible	7-pound bag	2	4	6	8

Bulk Items

Food Item	Notes & Tips	Unit	1	2	3	4
gluten-free rolled oats		cup	0.33	0.66	1	1.33
chia seeds	optional for legal cheat	cup	1	2	3	4
unsalted cashews		cup	0.5	1	1.5	2
raw pumpkin seeds		cup	0.25	0.5	0.75	1
raw almonds		cup	0.5	0.75	1	1.25
chopped dates	or 4/8/12/16 large pitted	tablespoon	4	8	12	16
golden raisins	optional if you can't find them	cup	0.5	1	1.5	2
quinoa		cup	1	2	3	4

Food Item	Notes & Tips	Unit	# of People on Detox			
			1	2	3	4
wild rice		cup	0.5	1	1.5	2
green or red lentils		pound	0.5	1	1.5	2

Miscellaneous

Food Item	Notes & Tips	Unit	1	2	3	4
liquid stevia		bottle	1	1	2	2
organic butter	unsalted	tablespoon	2	4	6	8
organic coconut oil		tablespoon	4	8	12	16
organic cinnamon		tablespoon	1	1	2	2
cumin		teaspoon	1	2	3	4
extra-virgin olive oil		cup	0.5	1	1.5	2
vegetable broth	no sodium, if bought canned	quart	1	2	3	4
real maple syrup		tablespoon	3	6	9	12
red-wine vinegar	raw if possible	tablespoon	3	6	9	12
raw apple cider vinegar		small bottle	1	1	1	1
dried thyme		teaspoon	1	2	3	4
nutritional or brewer's yeast						
cayenne	optional for Crunchy Avocado Salad	tablespoon	1	1	2	2
Spike seasoning (salt-free variety) or other extremely low-sodium seasoning		bottle	1	1	1	1
sprouted flax	see Resources page for GSG sprouted flax coupon					
organic protein product (any type)	see Resources page for GSG protein product coupon					
inexpensive citrus juicer (from discount store)	optional, but will help if making lemonade legal cheat					

:::: RECIPES::::

BLACK AND GREEN SALAD

Makes 5 one-cup servings

DRESSING:

1 heaping tablespoon grated lime zest

¼ cup fresh lime juice

¼ cup extra-virgin olive oil

2 teaspoons real maple syrup

1–2 teaspoons salt-free seasoning, such as Spike (optional)

SALAD:

1 cup quinoa, rinsed well (soak for a few minutes, then drain in a fine strainer)

2 cups water

1 can black beans (12 oz.), rinsed well (or ⅔ cup dry beans rinsed well and then simmered in 2 cups water for 2 hours)

2 medium tomatoes, diced

4 green onions, chopped (including most of the green part)

½ cup chopped fresh cilantro

Whisk together lime zest and juice, olive oil, maple syrup, and optional seasoning in a serving bowl. Simmer the quinoa in water uncovered for about 10 minutes. Turn off the heat, cover, and let stand 10 minutes. Strain any excess water, then add the quinoa to the dressing and toss well. Stir in the remaining ingredients (beans, tomatoes, green onions, cilantro). Serve warm, or chill in fridge.

BREAKFAST OATMEAL

Makes 1 serving

If you dislike oatmeal, you may wish to substitute another whole, cooked grain.

1 cup water

½ cup organic regular (not instant) rolled oats
(Bob's Red Mill and King Arthur Flour make this,
and you can optionally buy gluten-free oats,
although oats are naturally low in gluten)

pinch of cinnamon (optional)

few drops liquid stevia (optional)

Bring water to a boil, then add oats. Reduce heat and simmer 10 to 12 minutes. Add cinnamon and stevia if desired.

CLASSIC GREEN SMOOTHIE

Makes 2 quarts

The way I have written the recipe relies on your paying attention to the amount of blended water, greens, and fruit in the markings on the blender jar. I wrote it this way because greens are highly variable in size. "Handfuls" are similarly imprecise. If you wish to make it your own way, you can. The basic proportions I use are ⅓ water, ⅓ greens, and ⅓ fruit. The idea is to maximize the amount of greens and minimize the fruits to your own tastes. And one more note: the first four days of this recipe only call for the first four steps.

1. Start with 2½ cups of water/ice in the blender.

2. Add any three of these greens on any given day: mustard greens, beet tops, dandelion greens, spinach, collards, kale, romaine, mixed spring greens, cabbage, and chard.

3. Optionally add 1½ to 2 scoops organic, raw, vegan protein powder and 2 to 3 tablespoons sprouted flax. (See your Resources page. These are optional "nice to haves" to make the smoothies more sustaining, like a complete meal, with heart- and brain-healthy essential fatty acids.)

4. Blend until liquid comes to the 5- to 5½-cup line (add more greens if necessary to reach this line when blended).

5. To the remaining green smoothie mixture in the blender jar, add apples, frozen mixed berries, and/or bananas to the 7- to 8-cup line.

CRUNCHY AVOCADO SALAD

Makes 3 to 4 one-cup servings

2 whole avocados

3 Roma tomatoes, chopped (or 1 to 2 large regular tomatoes,
but Romas hold up better in the salad)

½ cup raw almonds, soaked overnight and drained,
coarsely chopped

1 to 2 stalks celery, finely chopped

1 green onion, diced

¼ cup cilantro, chopped

1 tablespoon fresh lemon juice

Spike (salt-free variety) or extremely low-sodium seasoning, to taste

1 to 2 tablespoons nutritional yeast (or brewer's yeast)

pinch of cayenne to taste (optional)

Chop 1 avocado. Toss all other ingredients, and add the chopped avocado to the portion for today's lunch (save the other avocado and chop just before adding it to tomorrow's portion, so that it doesn't turn brown).

CUCUMBER-TOMATO SALAD

Makes 7 one-cup servings

2 organic cucumbers

2 ripe organic tomatoes

½ small red onion (do *not* double this if expanding recipe for 2 to 3 people)

¼ cup apple cider vinegar

fresh basil or cilantro, to taste (optional)

Chop all ingredients and mix together well.

Note: A GreenSmoothieGirl reader said that lime juice and cilantro substituted for the apple cider vinegar and basil is delicious! If you do this, make sure to make these substitutions on your shopping list.

HOT PINK BREAKFAST SMOOTHIE

Makes 1 quart

1½ cups coconut liquid/water/juice (from a young coconut or a can, found in almost any food store; *not* coconut milk)

2 tablespoons chunk organic raw beet, peeled

1 large organic carrot, scrubbed

¼ cup unsalted cashews

2 tablespoons chopped dates *OR* 2 large pitted dates

12 ounces frozen organic strawberries

Purée all but the strawberries in a high-speed blender for 90 seconds. Add the strawberries and blend until smooth, about 90 seconds. Serve immediately.

LENTIL SOUP

Makes 10 one-cup servings

This makes a very large batch, so if you are not doing the detox with a buddy, you can share with your family or friends—or freeze it for later use after the detox. You can add sea salt to your family's portion, but remember that you are seeking very low sodium on the detox.

½ pound green or red lentils

½ cup wild rice, rinsed well

3 large yellow onions, diced

2 cloves garlic, minced

2 tablespoons organic coconut oil

1 teaspoon salt-free or extremely low-sodium herbal seasoning, or more to taste

1 teaspoon dried thyme

1 teaspoon cumin

4 stalks celery, diced

3 carrots, diced

1 quart vegetable broth (no-sodium, if you buy canned)

1 6-ounce can tomato sauce

2 teaspoons red-wine vinegar

Cover lentils and rice with boiling water and let sit for 15 minutes, then drain. In a large stock pot, sauté the onions and garlic with the coconut oil and seasonings until the vegetables are tender. Add the carrots and celery and sauté another 5–10 minutes. Add the vegetable broth, tomato sauce, and lentils and rice. Bring to a boil, reduce heat, and simmer 1 hour. Add vinegar and serve.

Tip: This soup tastes even better the second and third days. I suggest you make it a day ahead of time, if possible.

PURPLE HEAVEN

Makes 4 one-cup servings

SALAD:

2 cups shredded green cabbage

2 cups shredded red cabbage

½ cup golden raisins (optional, if you can't find them, but they add something very special)

¼ cup raw pumpkin seeds

DRESSING:

2 tablespoons real maple syrup

2 tablespoons extra-virgin olive oil

2 tablespoons red-wine vinegar

1 clove garlic, minced

Toss salad ingredients in a large bowl. Blend dressing ingredients and add to cabbage mixture.

:::: DETOXING YOUR BODY, :::: MIND, AND SPIRIT

Although the focus of the detox is on food, purifying the body to align physical health with higher emotional and spiritual health is often one of its purposes. This 7-Day Detox is mostly, but not entirely, about the fuel you're choosing. And it's an experiment in noticing how the fuel you choose changes your energetics on every level.

However, because one week of significant effort, while very helpful, obviously isn't enough for you to live in a qualitatively different state forever, I have some suggestions beyond the food realm for you to be thinking about.

I want to encourage you to consider your high-vibration life a journey rather than a destination. But you'll complete this book, and the 7-Day Detox, with awareness and tools to dramatically improve your life, now and in your future.

Four simple ideas I'd love you to consider will also help you "detox" your emotional reaction to life, if you make them practices:

1. Filter your thoughts to be accepting, noncritical, and even loving to others—even those you've felt critical of in the past or who have wronged you. Experiment with showing compassion, even when it is not "deserved," to yourself and to others.

2. Take note of your negative moods and negative thoughts. When you notice you don't feel good for some reason, scan your body. Notice where the negative feeling resides. (Your heart, belly, shoulders, or head might be uncomfortable. Where do you feel it?)

3. Be patient and noncritical of yourself as you observe, but become more mindful of when you're uncomfortable and what the reason is. Experiment with self-talk using positive words and memories of

wins, big and small, in your life to reverse any downward-spiraling, low-vibe thought patterns. (For example, "I can do hard things. I've done hard things before.")

My tennis teammate Christine is popular on the team and a favorite doubles partner because of her consistently positive talk during a match. She told us once that she repeats positive mantras to herself throughout a match, such as "My serve is awesome!" She said to us, "If you tell it to yourself enough times, the body believes it!" Reminding yourself, as you detox, what a wonderful process you're serving your body, mind, and spirit with is immeasurably helpful.

4. Become more aware, when you make a mistake, of how you find excuses or blame others. Practice immediately being accountable, rather than parsing and discussing blame, and see how that feels.

The week that I wrote this, I'd said something snarky in an e-mail thread with my very large family. I went to bed feeling uncomfortable, and sleep eluded me. Early the next morning, I wrote a text to my family that started like this:

"I woke up wanting to be accountable for what I said yesterday, so I wanted to be clear about that and tell you that I'm sorry."

What came back from my siblings in the text thread was "Thank you" and "I love you"—very different from the cold pricklies I was getting the night before after my barbed message that many read. Even better, my guilty feelings, which earlier in my life I'd covered up with anger and blaming, dissipated, and my comfortable, peaceful Optimal ViQ returned.

I highly recommend taking immediate responsibility whenever you can—even if you don't feel it's quite your "fault." This quickly releases negative vibrations; it disarms people, and they feel closer to you and safer with you; it energizes relationships that may be strained; and it shows you to be rational, reasonable, and fair.

These are character traits all of us are attracted to. So, how can it be bad to just say, "I did thus-and-such, and I'm so sorry. It won't happen again, and please forgive me?"

The cost of doing this is lower than you think. If you practice "swallowing your pride" regularly, you don't choke on it.

:   :   :   :   :

Detoxing your colon, liver, and kidneys goes a long way toward your Optimal ViQ, but there are bad vibes hiding in other places that need cleansing. When you let go of negative feelings, you're moving along the continuum toward a more beautiful life, attracting more of the good and less of the bad.

May your journey be instructive, and may you have opportunities along the way to uplift others. May you always live in the high frequencies and be a powerful energetic force for good. Namaste.

A NOTE ON REFERENCES

Find links to all the research and studies referred to in this book at www.GreenSmoothieGirl.com/VibeResources.

ACKNOWLEDGMENTS

I want to express gratitude to the people who made this book possible. At Simon & Schuster: Michele Martin, Diana Ventimiglia, Cindy Ratzlaff, Karen Adelson, John Vairo, Lisa Litwack, Paul Metcalf, Alexandre Su, and Emma Powers, and my agents Celeste Fine and Sarah Passick, for your efforts to bring this book to market—and for believing in me, and this concept, in the first place.

To ten years of GreenSmoothieGirl followers online, the wind under my wings: you remind me that my work matters in your quality of life. I listen and try to serve every day.

Nothing I've done in ten years online and fifteen books would have been possible without the GreenSmoothieGirl team, and my longtime editor, Deb Tokarewich, who has worked on fourteen of my fifteen books. They edited, gave honest feedback, contributed ideas, made the graphics, and ran the show while I was busy writing, plus helped me film and build the beautiful resources we put together for our readers.

Thank you to my best friend and CMO, Kristin Matthews, and to Nikki Hunter, Jason Ruona, Jamison Stokdyk, Chad Gravallese, Annie Epperley, Sue Squire, Kami Hall, Caroline Lowman, Amy Jensen, and Malia Halstvedt.

To my four beautiful children: Kincade, Emma, Mary Elizabeth, and Tennyson, I love you. And to Daphne, who died right after I handed off the manuscript of this book, but who sat in my lap as I wrote all 90,000 words, and even did yoga and t'ai chi outside in the sunshine and fresh air with me, for our "five-in-one" exercises in this book we made for you in video form. You raised my vibration, as furry family members do for their humans, the world over.